Quantum Physics

A New Scientific Knowledge Brought to Light

(The Secrets of New Scientific Knowledge Made Uncomplicated and Practical)

Maurice Johnson

Published By **Ryan Princeton**

Maurice Johnson

Quantum Physics: A New Scientific Knowledge Brought to Light (The Secrets of New Scientific Knowledge Made Uncomplicated and Practical)

ISBN 978-1-988842-09-7

No part of this guidebook shall be reproduced in any form without permission in writing from the publisher except in the case of brief quotations embodied in critical articles or reviews.

Legal & Disclaimer

The information contained in this book is not designed to replace or take the place of any form of medicine or professional medical advice. The information in this book has been provided for educational & entertainment purposes only.

The information contained in this book has been compiled from sources deemed reliable, and it is accurate to the best of the Author's knowledge; however, the Author cannot guarantee its accuracy and validity and cannot be held liable for any errors or omissions. Changes are periodically made to this book. You must consult your doctor or get professional medical advice before using any of the suggested remedies, techniques, or information in this book.

Table Of Contents

Chapter 1: What Is Quantum Physics?

They have a study of quantum physics is taken into consideration one among technology's more modern disciplines, however it has its roots in centuries of gathered expertise. Physics itself is a massive clinical field, encompassing the test of nature, depend, and energy. It includes research and assessment of ways all rely acts and reacts, which incorporates thru moderate, sound, kinetic energy, magnetism, and the conduct of the atom. Quantum physics seeks to reply questions about don't forget range and power on its smallest, maximum important tiers and broadest, most standard degrees. Looking on the history of the elements at play in contemporary quantum physics offers perception into how those requirements form the sector of test we see in recent times.

Quantum physics grew from the same old beginnings of classical physics, which has been studied due to the fact the Sumerians first located chisel to tablet. The easy machines that anyone found out approximately in grade college are examples of classical physics in motion. And we're excessive fine that everybody's heard the story of Archimedes coming across quantity and displacement in his historical Grecian tub. The fact is, physics is all spherical us, all the time. Gravity is what's keeping you from floating away right now. Physics keep your car walking and, on the road, and your headlights illuminating your manner. Without physics, we wouldn't be capable of enjoy the manner of lifestyles that we do in the present day-day age. Since we're right here to speak approximately quantum physics, allow's get matters started out with a observe the origins of the region, starting with the number one atomic idea.

The Grandfather of Atomic Study

It's the atom itself that bureaucracy the basis for the specialized subject of quantum physics.

Although the atom changed into first defined in 4 hundred B.C. Via a Greek truth seeker named Democritus, it wasn't until 1803 that the primary scientific atomic idea grow to be superior thru British chemist John Dalton.

Dalton changed into a pioneer in predictive meteorology and the take a look at of genetic coloration blindness before shifting onto atomic chemistry. He released a theorem in 1808, which actual what he considered to be the five houses of the atom.

1Atoms can not be destroyed or divided

2All the atoms in a unmarried element are equal

threeAtoms of different factors have wonderful residences and weights

fourThe atoms of numerous elements can be jumbled in smooth numbers to form molecules (Dalton used the word "compounds")

5Atoms may be neither created nor destroyed; all depend will damage down in recoverable, unchanged atoms.

Using the ones standards, Dalton may additionally create the primary rudimentary periodic desk. It contained superb six elementshydrogen, oxygen, nitrogen, carbon, sulfur, and phosphorushowever showed the relative weights of an atom of every element based on hydrogen having a cost of 1 (1). Dalton gave the scientific community a business enterprise basis on which to construct the field we now understand as quantum physics.

In truth, little or no has modified in the over centuries because of the fact Dalton first posted his atomic concept in a ebook called A New System of Chemical Philosophy.

The extremely good massive edit in his precept in the -plus centuries even as you keep in mind that its e-book is that we now understand that the atom isn't the smallest unit of rely; an atom's character additives also can be visible and measured. We furthermore now understand that an atom can be cut up, and we've the generation to achieve this.

Avogadro and His Gases

Using the paintings of Dalton as his basis, Italian scientist Amedeo Avogadro began his groundbreaking have a have a examine of the behavior of gases. Avogadro believed there might be a flaw in one of Dalton's theories on this topic. While there has been no flaw in Dalton's bodily paintings, there has been a small mistake in his interpretation of the way water absorbed carbon dioxide, nitrogen, and one of a kind numerous gases. Dalton believed that the water behaved in another way given the attention of the gases. In comparison, Avogadro can also want to move on to show that it become as an alternative the atomic weight of the gases that created the differing reactions.

Avogadro's maximum first rate legacy in the place of quantum physics is his namesake huge variety, seen right here:

6.02214076 × 1023 = 1 mole

This equation represents the amount of debris (atoms, molecules, ions, and so forth.) which can be contained inner a substance held at a particular amount, pressure, and temperature. This unit is now known as a mole and is diagnosed as an SI Unit with the photo mol. Avogadro theorized and ultimately proved that that may be a ordinary reality that governs all gases and that an same volume of any fuel on the same temperature and strain will consist of this large style of debris, regardless of atomic weight. A stunning element about Avogadro's equation is that it may be used to convert atoms to moles and moles to atoms, primarily based on what know-how the scientist already possesses. This is due to the truth the molar weight of a substance and the atomic weight of the substance are the equal. For example:

Water molecules are made from hydrogen atoms and one oxygen atom

The blended molecular weight of a water molecule is 18.1/2 amu (atomic mass gadgets)

Therefore, a mole of water weighs 18.Half of grams, expressed as g/mol.

Being capable of calculate the atomic weights and convert backward and forward from mass to molar devices makes it that a lot a lot less complicated for scientists to art work with large numbers and comprehend the massive variety of atoms that make up each recognized substance.

Let's check a calculation wherein we recognize the atomic weight but want to calculate the large style of atoms interior a stated sample of carbon, which has an atomic weight of 12 amu.

Carbon is often used as the usual in the direction of which all excellent atomic weights are measured due to the reality this is the substance upon which Avogadro built his equation. Therefore:

12 grams of carbon-12 have an atomic amount same to at the least one mol (6.022×1023)

To calculate the molar weight or molar amount of a few other substance, without a doubt plug inside the range that you do recognize and the variables that you don't; the ones equations look like this:

If you already know the amount of moles (x) but want to calculate the form of atoms (y), use this equation:

x moles·6.022×1023 = y atoms

1 mole

Reversing the calculation above, it's far possible to convert a few atoms to a molar amount by dividing it with the useful aid of Avogadro's massive range.

If the style of atoms (x) however need to calculate the style of moles (y), use this form of the equation:

x atoms

6.022×1023 atoms = y moles

1mole

This can be written without a fragment inside the denominator by multiplying the variety of atoms via the reciprocal of Avogadro's variety:

x atoms·1 mole = y moles

6.022×1023

Because it's so useful in calculating atomic content material and molar weights, Avogadro's wide range is frequently known as Avogadro's Constant. Avogadro's Constant is used to calculate the amount of a substance internal any measurable area.

It's particularly beneficial in letting scientists communicate big numbers of particles with one SI Unit.

Constructing the Atom

Without walking expertise of the form of the atom, how would it be possible to have a study its conduct and decide its houses? Simply put, it wouldn't be, and so it's important to recognize the artwork of the scientists who labored to plan the primary models of an atom as we apprehend them in recent times. These early fashions weren't quality however gave the researchers who got here later a better expertise of methods the ones tiny particles of rely wide variety artwork and engage.

One of the earliest fashions of the atom modified into created with the aid of British physicist J.J. Thomson in 1904, called the 'plum pudding' model. Thomson is credited with coming across the negatively-charger atomic sub-particle now referred to as the electron. Thomson observed out that for an atom to be held together, there have to moreover be a counteracting fantastic price. Named for the famous British dessert of bread pudding with raisins, the plum pudding version of the atom showed a place of positivity (the pudding) embedded with awful electrons (the raisins). Thomson have become on the right song, but the model of the atom wasn't quite there however.

The next advancement within the going for walks model of an atom modified into thru the studies of Ernest Rutherford and his college university college students Hans Geiger and Ernest Marsden, in 1911. The Geiger-Marsden experiments concerned bombarding thin gold foil with alpha rays. The university college students and Rutherford determined that handiest approximately ninety% of the rays went through the foil. The different percent changed into deflected, critical the scientists to accept as actual with that some issue was inflicting the deflection. In flip, this declaration encouraged them to the speculation that every atom actually had a center, or nucleus, that turned into capable of turning away the movement of alpha rays. The ensuing version became the number one cloud example of the atom, one with a nucleus with electrons floating in ordinary orbits, in place of randomly bouncing around, because the plum pudding model had portrayed.

In 1913, running with Danish physicist Niels Bohr, the version end up updated slightly to apprehend that the nucleus of the atom changed into manufactured from the subatomic particle now called the proton. The proton and the electron artwork together to maintain the atom at a impartial electric powered rate. The Rutherford-Bohr version is more normally surely referred to as the Bohr model. It's this illustration that the widespread majority of human beings, from the youngest of important faculty science university students to the most superior theoretical physicists, use and are acquainted with these days.

It wasn't till physicist and former Rutherford scholar James Chadwick positioned the neutron in 1932 that the whole photo of the atom came into interest. While the research changed into abruptly advancing within the difficulty of radioactivity (extra on that in a chunk), scientists were finding it hard to reconcile the atomic weights of factors based completely definitely upon the presence of protons and electrons. While the amount of protons in an atom defines its atomic extensive variety, the mass of the nucleus determines its atomic weight. So, in which have become the differential coming from? Chadwick theorized that there ought to be some exceptional particle in the nucleus affecting the atomic weight, but not the electric rate of the atom.

Using this speculation, Chadwick finished a chain of experiments the use of alpha and gamma radiation to show his theories. The results confirmed the exposure of a brand new subatomic particle, the neutron.

Neutrons are intermixed with protons within the nucleus of the atom and solved the puzzle of why atomic weights were no longer identical to atomic variety. This improvement inside the facts of the development of the atom earned Chadwick as Nobel Prize for

Physics in 1935 and forever modified the face of quantum physics.

Radioactivity, Isotopes, and Pioneering Research

The funny difficulty about the discovery of subatomic particles and the primary accurate models of the atom is that those upgrades got here past due in the game within the preliminary wave of trends in quantum physics.

The creation of these correct fashions, but, gave the scientists who located the capability to appearance lower again on the paintings of their predecessors and use their research to develop the arena of quantum physics with the useful resource of leaps and limits.

The art work of the earliest particle physicists isn't always something to be unnoticed. One of the maximum essential discoveries of the overdue 19th century is that of radioactivity.

French scientist Henri Becquerel, who may also artwork with Pierre and Marie Curie, have become experimenting with phosphorescent minerals when he stumbled upon what is going to be the primary recorded instance of spontaneous radioactivity at the same time as studying uranium salts. Spurred via the discovery of X-rays by the usage of way of his colleague Wilhelm Röntgen early in 1896, Becquerel speculated that uranium salts ought to characteristic in a good buy the identical way and concept he ought to harness the strength of their phosphorescence thru exposing them to vivid slight like sunlike.

What Becquerel may need to quickly find out is that he didn't want a slight supply to prompt the phosphorescence of the uranium salts. Coupled with studies on thorium, in addition to art work on polonium and radium being performed by way of way of the Curies, theories and evidence of natural radioactivity ought to snowball within the years fundamental as a good deal as the turn of the 20th century. Ironically sufficient, a colleague of Becquerel's father, both of whom have been furthermore early physicists, had almost through coincidence placed radioactivity nearly forty years previous to the more youthful Becquerel's findings.

That scientist, Frenchman Abel Niépce de Saint-Victor, come to be learning pictures and photosensitive processing materials at the equal time as he observed that uranium-based totally chemical compounds have to reveal photographic plates earlier than they had been subjected to slight-processing.

If he had been curious enough to transport one step further into why uranium had this effect on the ones photographic plates, he might have been the only to win the Nobel Prize for the invention.

Scientists have been capable of harness the power of radioactivity even before they really understood precisely what must be blamed for this behavior. Along with the discovery of x-rays, early artwork the usage of alpha, beta, and gamma rays modified into additionally underway. Researchers have been beginning to recognize the "how" of radioactivity and radiation, despite the fact that they didn't however recognize the "why." Using those rays grow to be a massive beautify in early quantum physics, and scientists like Becquerel, the Curies, Rutherford, and their students and cohorts have been able to make notable advances in their experimentation via using rays.

What those pioneering physicists did apprehend is that every atom of every element is in a regular usa of the usa of flux. The subatomic particles that make up an atom have to pass that allows you to produce the electromagnetic electricity critical to hold the atom together.

This motion produces waste strength, that is emitted within the form of radiation. Some factors are extra sturdy than others, and therefore require little electricity to keep their form. These factors have much less radioactivity, that is the degree for a manner a tremendous deal power, or radiation, an atom emits. Other factors, like radium, uranium, and thorium, are plenty a great deal less sturdy. They require a big quantity of atomic electricity to preserve their shape. Consequently, the ones elements have a better degree of radioactivity.

Using this expertise, scientists had been capable of begin concentrating this radiation. X-rays, of route, were decided to be beneficial in exposing pix hidden interior sturdy devices whilst combined with photographic processing. It changed into Rutherford who classified alpha, beta, and gamma rays, permitting his college college students to apply alpha radiation to finish the famous Geiger-Marsden experiments, which allowed them to hypothesize the proper nature of the empty region interior an atom. Rutherford named and labeled the sorts of radiation primarily based totally on their talents to penetrate one of a kind strong materials. Alpha radiation is made up of large, slower-shifting particles. Beta radiation is faster and product of slightly smaller particles than alpha radiation.

Gamma radiation consists of tiny, transferring particles. Because gamma rays supply little to no electric powered price, they are capable of penetrate most gadgets comfortably, no matter density or mass. There are, of direction, other forms of radiation; electromagnetic emissions like microwaves and infrared, ultraviolet, and seen mild also are labeled as radiation.

Radioactivity, the term coined by means of the use of Becquerel and made famous by using way of the Curies, is immediately related to the nucleus of the atom and its natural breakdown.

Once the discovery of radioactivity became made, it wasn't an lousy lot of a jump to discover precisely what delivered on it and what set some atoms other than others.

It might be every other Rutherford colleague, Frederick Soddy, who need to first hint at the lifestyles of isotopesvariations on the subatomic make-up of atoms of the same factors. As it appears, the nucleus of an atom, which incorporates protons and neutrons, may additionally have a variable form of neutrons, which affects the stableness of the nucleus. The result of this variable amount of neutrons are isotopes, which can be defined as top notch species of the atoms which make up and element.

In factors with excessive radioactive values, like uranium or thorium, isotopes are frequently volatile and regularly losing neutrons primary to rapid alternate and breakdown. Becquerel and Marie and Pierre Curie, whose pioneering research into those sorts of relatively radioactive substances, could also be some of the primary to apprehend that the heavy gamma radiation emitted have turn out to be additionally the purpose of terrible, irreversible mobile harm, which we apprehend now to be radiation poisoning. Becquerel died from the headaches of exceptional burns, later observed out to had been delivered approximately with the useful resource of his unprotected managing of uranium salts. Perhaps Pierre Curie can also have furthermore been taken via the use of radiation poisoning, had he no longer been killed in a carriage twist of fate in 1906. His lifestyles and clinical fulfillment had been cut tragically quick, however Marie carried on their paintings with the help in their daughter Irene till her very personal death from radiation-related leukemia in 1934.

She stays the incredible woman to have received Nobel prizes; the number one in Physics became for the Curies' paintings along Becquerel in 1903, and the second in Chemistry for her discovery of polonium and radium.

All elements have a diploma of radioactivity.

The studies published thru Becquerel, Rutherford, and the Curies brought about a much greater facts of the person of the atom, the way to degree radioactive decay, and a manner to use radiation appropriately and purposefully.

The discovery of the lifestyles of isotopes is what gave the world cellular x-ray machines, carbon-12 relationship, and in the long run, nuclear electricity and nuclear weapons.

This is all thanks to isotopes and their decay styles.

If you'll don't forget John Dalton's houses of an atom, he states explicitly that atoms cannot be created or destroyed. While we have the era to expose Dalton incorrect, he become moreover accurate on a crucial part of that assets. It's count itself that can't be created or destroyed, as examined in Antoine Lavoisier's 1789 Law of the Conservation of Mass.

Let's take a better check what occurs to depend inside the route of a chemical method or radioactive decay.

Conserving Matter, Energy, and Mass

There are legal hints that govern the whole thing we realize approximately bodily keep in mind and power, and people time-commemorated legal guidelines shape every the backbone and the limiting elements of physics in the course of the records of the issue.

The Law of the Conservation of Matter, additionally known as Conservation of Mass, states that irrespective of can be created or destroyed, simplest modified into every other form. The Law of Conservation of Energy states that energy can not be created or destroyed, best transferred or transformed. Together, those felony tips inform us the whole lot we need to understand about balancing chemical and bodily reactions, which includes radioactivity. These felony guidelines assist us understand that the entirety that exists and actions inside the bodily worldwide is crafted from some thing else; not anything is conjured out of nothing. The uncooked substances that make up all things are the tiniest subatomic debris and the electricity they emit.

When you want to observe the greater advanced requirements of quantum physics, it's essential to hold the ones prison tips within the again of your mind. Before the conservation laws were hypothesized, tested, and cemented, alchemy have emerge as a well-known workout, and relatively, alchemists had the right idea, no matter the fact that they in no manner did turn reason gold.

It is viable to convert one element into a few different, however whilst Soddy was growing the studies that triggered the discovery of isotopes, he additionally modified into essential in growing the Law of Radioactive Displacement. This law proved that an atom in active radioactive decay have to remodel into a few extraordinary element and that the modern-day element is decided thru the usage of whether or not or no longer or no longer the real element is emitting both alpha or beta radiation. Working in most instances with thorium (an isotope of radium), Soddy located that an atom that out of place neutrons via alpha decay should transmute to grow to be an element areas to the left at the periodic desk, and those that lost neutrons via beta decay would possibly transmute into an detail one place to the right on the table.

Polish-American physicist Kazimierz Fajans, working in Rutherford's laboratory in Manchester, England, additionally independently developed the same speculation at the same time as coming across the conduct of uranium; because of this, the Law of Radioactive Displacement is credited to every guys. Fajans is likewise credited with groundbreaking studies into the 1/2-life values of uranium.

A 1/2-life is the quantity of time it takes for an atom to break all of the manner right down to half of of its unique mass.

Therefore, after one half of of-existence, there can be 50% left; after half of-lives, there is probably 25% left, 3 will go away 12.Five%, and so forth.

Highly radioactive factors should have hundreds shorter 1/2 of of-lives than strong elements. But if we're speakme approximately each decay and conservation of depend, wherein does the rest of the atom's precise mass pass?

Let's take a look at an example that assist you to make easy the manner you think about the conservation of depend.

Imagine you're going to have a campfire.

You pile up your timber, moderate a wholesome, and your fireplace blazes up.

After multiple hours, you're all out of fuel, and you're left with a heap of ashes in which your pile of wood as soon as have grow to be. The wood is certainly long past, but if count number extensive variety cannot be created or destroyed, wherein did it go?

The pile of ashes isn't nearly similar in extent to the logs that you commenced with, so remember should had been destroyed, right? Wrongit's simply been transmuted. Think approximately the materials that make up a log of firewood; it includes natural compounds like cellulose, elemental vitamins, and water.

When those components are surrounded via airflow, which incorporates oxygen, nitrogen, and different atmospheric gases, and the chemical way of ignition and fireplace is applied, severa subjects begin to occur.

One of the number one bodily matters you may phrase even as you mild a campfire is which you'll pay interest sizzling and spot steam. The warmth of the hearth is changing the phase of the water molecules contained to your firewood, and the liquids have become gases. The recall that become water to start with contained within the log is the same quantity of depend, it's in reality been launched into the surroundings.

27

As your hearth burns, you'll begin to see greater modifications. The elements that make up the cellulose structures of the timber will begin to interrupt down into greater easy molecules and ultimately into its atomic components. The strong remnants can be gift inside the shape of ash, whose mass may be an awful lot smaller than the proper mass. That manner that the relaxation of the crucial composition of your campfire will have been launched into the surroundings because the gases discovered in steam and smoke.

Your equation started out out as essentially strong, with a small amount of liquid content fabric cloth and the atmospheric gases present to spark the chemical response of fire. In the forestall, maximum of the matter will have been converted into vaporous gases, leaving the solids elemental ashes behind. If you can lure and diploma the gases and add it to the mass of the ashes, you will find out them to be identical to the mass of timber and gases which you started with. You must keep in mind the equation like this:

Firewood + atmospheric gases + catalyst (in form) = atmospheric gases + ashes

This is obviously a simplified take a look at the regulation in query, however it gives you a valid basis for considering depend as a everyday.

The one in every of a type law we're concerned about in this phase is The Law of Conservation of Energy, so allow's start to consider that during vital terms, as well.

The Law of Conservation of Energy is one of the oldest tenets of the have a take a look at of physics. As a reminder, it states that power can not be created or destroyed however can trade forms. There is a caveat to this due to the reality it could simplest be set up in a closed machine in which the electricity can't be acted upon thru outdoor forces. Energy is available in numerous paperwork, which might be expressed as every capacity or kinetic. Potential energy is the strength this is being stored or built up internal matter number for destiny use.

In assessment, kinetic power is the strength that rely makes use of at the same time as it is lively or in motion. To visualize capability as opposed to kinetic power, do not forget a pendulum or a toddler on a swing. When the pendulum is at the best thing it may be, it's far showing functionality electricity. As quickly as the pendulum starts offevolved offevolved offevolved to swing, it's miles showing kinetic electricity.

All power can be classified as follows:

Mechanical: This is the power that is discovered in bodily items, and the entire of mechanical energy is the kinetic plus the potential strength.

A transferring object is the use of kinetic strength, making its functionality strength 0.

A resting item shifts the equation within the one-of-a-kind direction. An example of an item with a balance of kinetic and functionality strength is probably a car the use of up a steep hill. The vehicle is shifting, but now not at its pinnacle pace, this means that that it is not the usage of all of its ability energy.

Electromagnetic (Radiant): This is the form of power that refers to anything that locations off electromagnetic waves or mild, even non-visible spectrums like ultraviolet or infrared.

Electromagnetic strength also may be potential or kinetic, and this is probably exhibited in a few thing like a lightbulb and moderate transfer.

The ability energy is being held in the closed circuit. When the switch is flipped, the circuit opens, allowing energy to come to be kinetic, turning at the lightbulb, which similarly converts that electrical strength into mild and warmth. Microwaves, radio waves, and gamma rays are all additionally examples of electromagnetic energy.

Chemical: Chemical electricity is the strength used or launched finally of chemical tactics or reactions.

A terrific example of the capability and kinetic strength of a chemical way is a stick of dynamite.

The dynamite well-known capacity strength earlier than the application of the catalyst, in this case, hearth, and on the identical time because it explodes, it's far displaying unexpected and violent kinetic electricity. It also converts some of its functionality strength into sonic and thermal electricity, which we'll cowl in a 2nd. A a lot less explosive example of chemical energy in actual lifestyles is probably a disposable battery powering a toy or a plant using its chlorophyll, water, atmospheric gases, and radiant strength to create glucose to feed itself and oxygen to emit.

Sonic: Sonic power is, in fact, precisely what it 'sounds' likethis is the power of sound waves.

Sound waves can not exist in a vacuum; they have to have each other medium thru which to tour, which incorporates the air or water. Some right examples of sonic strength are the sound of your voice or track being done, or a sonic boom from a jet plane.

Thermal: Thermal electricity is the power of heat. Heat is produced via some of chemical manner, and it's far allocated among structures through convection, conduction, or direct transfer. Simply located, warmth is constantly in search of to excursion to wherein there can be a scarcity of warmth. Thermal energy is measured via finding the distinction inside the baseline temperature of the 2 systems.

Thermal electricity is also important in knowledge how chemical and mechanical strength is transferred among structures.

Nuclear: Nuclear energy is what is created whilst the center a part of the atom, the nucleus, is break up apart through both mechanical or chemical way. It takes a top notch deal of pressure to break apart the nucleus, and that strain is redirected into nuclear electricity, which may be harnessed for energy and to power engines.

Nuclear strength, as most humans apprehend, additionally may be contained in guns of mass destruction like bombs and warheads. One of the unlucky byproducts of nuclear electricity is the ensuing dangerous waste, which collects from the spent nuclear gasoline and will take an exceptionally long term to cycle via its last half-lives to turn out to be inactive.

Gravitational: Gravitational electricity is the force that keeps devices attracted to each. This best example of gravitational strength is the relationship the various solar and the planets or the Earth and the moon. Gravitational electricity, or pull, is also what keeps up recognition on the floor and now not flying off into place. Being able to understand gravitational energy is a crucial part of having the ability to check and recognize the physics of now not first-rate our planet however the solar gadget and past into deep area. Gravitational power can offer an cause of astronomical phenomena that we are capable of't see with our modern-day technology.

If nothing else, quantum physics is ready the relationship some of the devices in our universe, from the tiniest subatomic debris visible with our most precise microscopes to the maximum huge stars and astronomical our our bodies past the scope of our best telescopes. Now that you've have been given a piece of data and a primer on strength and remember, it's time to move without delay to a number of quantum physics' huge standards and groundbreaking discoveries. We'll start through taking a more in-depth examine the debris themselves and the way they flow into through the area.

Chapter 2: The De Broglie Equation

In the ultimate monetary ruin, we talked masses approximately the homes of atoms and the character of power. The subatomic particles that make up atoms and the conduct of these atoms are the focal point of quantum physics.

In this chapter, we're going to dive into the manner atoms and subatomic debris skip, how this movement can be measured and affected, and the effect that subatomic movement has on the examine of modern-day quantum physics.

Particle Theory

In order to apprehend particles, you must first recognize the mind of particle concept. The Particle Theory of Matter and the Particle Theory of Energy give us some ordinary truths about the tiniest portions of our global. These theories are the absolutes on which quantum physics is based totally definitely, so permit's go over the tenets that make up the Particle Theories.

The Particle Theory of Matter consists of 5 easy statements:

All rely is crafted from tiny particles, this first announcement seems obvious, as even "no longer anything" is manufactured from some problem. Still, with out putting this baseline, it's no longer feasible to assemble the relaxation of the particle precept and all unique theories that make up quantum physics.

All individual materials are composed of their very private type of rely, this precept is what lets in scientists to categorize acknowledged factors and understand whether or not or no longer newly placed substances are isotopes of previously recognized elements or capacity new factors.

All debris are constantly in motion-, this movement is crucial to preserve atomic bonds. If the debris that make up an atom have been to stop transferring abruptly, the atom might collapse.

The temperature at once affects how fast debris passThe warmer the particles, the faster they circulate. You can see this in an check as smooth as freezing a few water, then letting it thaw and swirling it round a pitcher at room temperature, and then boiling it. Steam movements masses faster than ice! Cold debris will slow all the way right down to hold electricity; heat debris have greater electricity to dissipate.

All debris show off attraction, the electric fee carried via atoms and molecules method that every one particles are looking to connect with exceptional like-minded debris. It is the ones bonds that link atoms into elements and factors into compounds.

Knowing these five tenets of the Particle Theory of Matter will help you similarly apprehend our subsequent fundamental of quantum physics, and that's the Particle Theory of Energy.

This concept is sometimes called the Kinetic Particle Theory, and it explains and lays down the ground regulations for the behaviors of particles at precise temperatures and incredible states of depend.

Kinetic Particle Theory lists the following traits of rely in its differing states:

Solid: Matter is in a robust nation whilst it's far at a temperature that does not allow its particles to transport freely. The debris in solids are arranged tightly together in a normal pattern, and they cannot bypass spherical; instead, they basically vibrate inside the vicinity they're allocated. There isn't any room maximum of the debris to permit for some other motion. Matter in a stable nation holds its very own form because of the strength of the bonds among debris.

Liquid: Matter in a liquid usa is depend that is at a temperature that allows the debris to spread out and take in extra area. In a liquid us of a, the debris are not constrained to a very good pattern.

They have more space in amongst them and might drift greater freely. These debris also are shifting quicker and extra inconsistently than they had been in a sturdy state.

Matter in a liquid u . S . A . Can not keep its form.

Rather, it takes the form of its area.

Gas: Matter in a gaseous nation is depend that has been heated to the thing of boiling or evaporation.

The temperature is excessive enough to permit the debris to place themselves out in a random sample and glide freely. If restricted, the debris will take the form of their box, and if unrestricted, they will assimilate with the environment. Particles in a gaseous nation are the fastest shifting and most erratic of all debris.

The temperature at which depend becomes sturdy, liquid, or gasoline is depending at the substance.

Water (H2O) will become strong at 0* Celsius and becomes a gasoline at 100°C. Another common substance, isopropyl alcohol (C3H8O), doesn't freeze until it reaches -89°C however additionally will become a fuel at a lower temperature than water.

The boiling thing of trade for isopropyl is 80.Four° C.

Every element and compound have its very non-public set of temperatures which have an effect on its u . S . A . Of matter.

It's critical to recognize the levels of be counted and the houses that accompany them, but it's also crucial to comprehend the thermal growth that underlies the ones modifications of state. Thermal enlargement does now not growth the mass of the substance or its debris.

You may want to have the same amount of ice, water, and steam as you started out with. What thermal growth does increase is the amount of area most of the debris on your substance. This growth is what allows the particles to boom their tempo and level of hobby. Another object of notice approximately the idea of thermal increase is whilst a gas has reached its maximum entropy diploma however is contained and does no longer have room to hold growing, the following physical pressure is pressure. That is why aerosol cans and distinctive fuel-filled devices shouldn't be subjected to excessive heat.

With no room left to transport, the ensuing rise in strain can result in an explosion.

Phase adjustments rise up thru a few chemical strategies. Gases are produced via each boiling or evaporation. Boiling, opposite to big belief, isn't clearly temperature set up. The crucial difference amongst boiling and evaporation is that boiling calls for lively input from an strength supply, which encompass a warm range burner beneath a tea kettle. The water will begin to boil, and steam may be released. In evaluation, evaporation ought to upward push up even as an open saucepan is disregarded on a countertop. Over time, the most lively (most excited) of the water molecules within the pan ought to "get away" from the floor into the surroundings.

When depend actions from a gaseous to a liquid us of a, it is thru the manner of condensation genuinely, the particles are converting lower returned from big erratic motion to a greater condensed circumstance.

Condensation takes region while the temperature lowers to a degree in which the particles can not preserve the quantity of movement they show off even as in a gaseous country. When the temperature lowers even in addition, liquids start to freeze or solidify into their sturdy states.

The opposite of this manner is solids melting into drinks.

Both melting and boiling arise whilst a substance reaches its latent temperature or has been plied with the proper amount of latent warm temperature. This is calculated with the beneficial aid of methods an entire lot energy desires to be accomplished to the substance to start the way of melting or boiling.

Instead of melting and boiling, you will likely every now and then see the terms "latent warm temperature of fusion" (melting) and "latent warm temperature of vaporization" (boiling).

There are two outliers to the Kinetic Particle Theory: The chemical approach of sublimation and the life of the fourth u . S . A . Of rely known as plasma. Sublimation is the change of rely immediately from the strong segment to the gasoline segment, surely skipping the liquid section. The incredible example of common sublimation is called "dry ice," this is frozen carbon dioxide (CO_2). When it starts offevolved offevolved to melt, it doesn't have a liquid us of a; it will become an evaporating gasoline proper now. This reaction can be hastened thru putting the dry ice in room temperature water. Dry ice is beneficial for transport and storing frozen objects because of its excessive capability to emit cold, and it's extensively implemented for pc snap shots like fog machines and Halloween decorations due to its functionality to fashionable.

Plasma is a piece of a ordinary idea to provide an reason behind.

The so-known as fourth nation of depend takes place at the identical time as debris are stripped in their electric fee, inflicting them to act in a completely erratic fashion.

Plasma is regularly taken into consideration to be a gas, however it doesn't behave within the identical way as a gas; plasma debris do not preserve even area amongst them, and that they don't have a cohesive enchantment.

These particles react efficiently to an electric powered price, this is why commonplace programs of plasma are neon or fluorescent lights and plasma televisions.

Now that we've laid the basics of particle and strength idea, it's time to talk about precisely how the ones particle characteristic and float. With those ground rules in thoughts, we're going to begin taking a better have a look at how the ones tiny debris make their manner through the universe, one wave at a time.

Wave Theory

We've all been to the seashore and have seen waves rolling into the shore or dropped a pebble right into a puddle and watched the water ripple out from in which the pebble broke the floor. We recognize this movement, but have you ever ever stopped to consider how and why those waves exist? What about thinking about those waves on the tiniest scale? What makes a wave a wave?

Waves are widely labeled into schooling, mechanical and electromagnetic, and we'll check those classifications in a bit on the equal time as.

Before we communicate about what makes waves special, allow's first observe what makes waves similar. We already understand that all particles are in movement all the time, even in a stable country. A wave takes place at the identical time as the ones debris begin to flow into in an observable, measurable, often predictable way. A wave cannot rise up without the outdoor effect of different forces upon the natural motion of the particles. However, a wave is NOT a particle.

A wave is energy in motion and does not private any mass.

Mechanical waves are a top instance of this. Mechanical waves are waves that flow materials and sound, however they want to have a medium via which to bypass; mechanical waves can't exist in a vacuum. Mechanical waves want to furthermore be created through manner of an outdoor forcethey do no longer display up spontaneously.

Using the example of a pebble dropped right right into a puddle, what motives the waves? The water, crafted from H2O molecules, is in a liquid country, which means the particles are transferring freely and taking up the form of the puddle. Those molecules are though bonded to each other, and on the surface of the puddle, the energy they may be the usage of to live linked effects in ground tension.

When that surface anxiety is broken through the mass of the pebble, that electricity (which, bear in mind, cannot be created, or destroyed) need to transport someplace, and so it's miles transformed into wave strength. The top (or amplitude) of these waves may be determined by way of the usage of the rate of the pebble, which in flip is probably determined with the useful resource of the peak and pressure at which it changed into dropped.

This also can even have an impact at the frequency of the waves, it truely is measured in how many waves skip a tough and fast factor in a hard and fast quantity of time, i.E., waves ordinary with 2d.

The 2d sort of waves are electromagnetic waves, and this category of waves consists of all spectrums of mild, x-rays, and gamma radiation.

Electromagnetic waves are manufactured from herbal electricity, and it is the amplitude and frequency of those waves that outline what shape of electricity it's far. Electromagnetic power does not need a physical medium to journey thru; as we understand, mild and one in all a type waves can excursion thru the vacuum of area.

Light electricity is break up into a large spectrum starting from ultraviolet thru seen slight and completing with infrared. The scale is based at the wavelength (frequency) of this energy. Light power falls inside the center of the electromagnetic wavelength scale, which starts offevolved offevolved with shortwave cosmic waves and culminates with longwave radio transmissions. The scale measures these waves in wavelengths and nanometers and is going from shortest wavelength to longest, like this:

Cosmic waves, Gamma rays, X-rays, Ultraviolet (UV) rays, Visible mild spectrum (violet, indigo, blue, inexperienced, yellow, orange, purple), Infrared, Microwave, Radar, Shortwave broadcast radio, FM radio, Analog Television, AM radio, Longwave broadcast radio.

We don't do not forget it, however waves are all spherical us at any given time. Most of these rays are mainly innocent, however scientists observed classes from the early days of on foot with x-rays and radiation that there can be harmful element effects of sure varieties of electromagnetic waves. It didn't take prolonged to give you easy, sensible answers to those exposure troubles, it is why to this modern, radiology technicians will wear and offer their sufferers lead-lined shields and aprons to save you any tissue damage from needless touch with x-rays. It's moreover why scientists and researchers put on shielding suits and gloves while working with drastically radioactive materials.

Waves are important in the workings of the universe. Without waves, we wouldn't have radio, tv, or microwave ovens. We wouldn't be able to speak with human beings at the opportunity factor of the place, or maybe with our astronauts in location. Waves are responsible for every coloration, tint, and hue of coloration that lighting fixtures our international and the mild that reaches us from the sun.

Scientists furthermore now recognize that gravitational waves are real and measurable, adding to our well-known understanding of waves and the manner the smallest and biggest quantities of our universe engage.

It can be hard to wrap your mind throughout the concept of waves as topics that exist but don't have mass. Instead of considering what they aren't, count on greater about what they areimperative,   transferring,   shipping structures. Without waves, we might have no lifestyles-giving slight from the solar and wouldn't have the capability to talk to each one-of-a-kind. Waves are vital and top notch. Now that we've discovered the basics within the lower back of particle and waves, we're going to study a idea that ties together those requirements and offers us a more records of the big picture of physics by way of further analyzing the tiniest elements.

de Broglie's Hypothesis of Particles and Waves

French physicist Louis de Broglie (who changed into also the seventh Duc de Broglie) came to prominence inside the mid to past due 1920s for his pioneering paintings on wave-particle duality that we'll be discussing at length in this segment. De Broglie grew up with a love of military history and rhetoric, and his first higher diploma come to be in the humanities.

He might glide right now to check and get hold of degrees in mathematics and physics and end up called a prolific learner and exemplary scholar.

In 1914, de Broglie entered into the French army to serve in World War I.

During this provider, he modified into stationed in Paris and assigned to boom, hold, and characteristic radio transmission devices, maximum famously, the handiest established at the Eiffel Tower.

He can also want to moreover be a few of the first to help installation radio communications device in submarines.

It turn out to be this enjoy with radio waves that ignited de Broglie's previous casual hobby in wave movement and behavior. When he turned into released from the army in 1919, de Broglie may additionally need to start task wave and particle experiments in his brother Maurice (additionally a physicist) laboratory. In 1924, he launched his seminal art work on the venture, Recherches sur l. A.

Théorie des quanta, or Research at the Theory of the Quanta.

His precept stated that "any shifting particle or item has an related wave.".

He based totally his hypothesis on his research of the artwork of Planck and Einstein, who have been undertaking giant research into the homes of slight strength and wave-particle duality.

The wave-particle duality idea have been developed to offer an motive behind the conduct of gadgets on a quantum scale.

de Broglie modified into interested in taking the wave-particle idea all of the way down to the quantum degree to decipher the hobby he became seeing in electrons.

He suspected that they've been behaving a bargain inside the same way as Einstein had tested mild to act while he theorized the life of photons.

Certain that electrons had been moreover appearing as and visiting in waves, de Broglie and his colleagues set about finding a manner to show the speculation.

The resulting studies led the scientists to the problem of our subsequent segment, de Broglie's Equation.

de Broglie's Equation

The de Broglie equation is an variant of some of Planck and Einstein's earlier equations explaining the conduct of mild inside the shape of photons. Using artwork performed thru George Paget Thomson on diffracted cathode rays and experiments on electron conduct now known as the Davisson-Germer research, de Broglie end up capable of finish that particles can and do, in reality, act as waves.

This is the equation he created to provide an cause for and calculate that conduct:

$\lambda = h/mv$

In this equation, the Greek image lambda represents the wavelength, h is Planck's ordinary (of which we are able to speak the development in a later financial disaster), m is the mass of the transferring particle, and v is consultant of the particle's velocity.

de Broglie's equation is used to show that particles exhibit the identical particle-wave duality as light.

The equation additionally serves to expose that wavelengths trade over the years a distance, as their initial energy shifts from ability to kinetic and lower back to capacity.

Have you ever seen a rhythmic gymnastics primary usual performance?

The gymnasts often use big, extended ribbons to create lovely visible outcomes whilst they complete their physical games. But the ones ribbons can illustrate the loss of electricity over the existence of a wave, even without de Broglie's famous equation. You can recreate this test at home with a period of ribbon.

Taking your ribbon, maintain it by way of the bring about one hand, horizontally to the ground. By doing this, you're developing the plane alongside which your waves will adventure. Now flow into your hand up and down in a fluid motion to create the amplitude of your wave. You will study that the waves are extra common in the direction of the deliver in their strength (your hand) then they are at the prevent of the ribbon. This is due to the fact they lose electricity over the years, and the wavelength begins to increase.

The amplitude may also even begin to decrease.

You've correctly proven why and how de Broglie's equation calculates the commonplace wave motion of a particle over the years.

For his art work, de Broglie changed into provided the Nobel Prize in Physics in 1929, and Davisson and Germer could also attain the award in 1937 for their functionality to reveal the hypothesis of their laboratories. De Broglie went directly to pioneer, increase, and check hypotheses on neutrino mass, thermodynamics, and duality in the legal guidelines of physics and nature, but it's miles his equation for which remains the best mentioned.

Chapter 3: The Schrödinger Equation

About technological information is the clinical technique itself. If you take into account any of your junior immoderate technological understanding instructions, you'll without a doubt maintain in thoughts analyzing that the idea of all era is being capable of produce documented, measurable, repeatable, tangible results. Maybe you had a instructor who've end up a stickler for correctly stored lab notebooks.

For the men and women who revolutionized the field of quantum physics, carefully notating and documenting all their studies allowed them to create particular papers and books, giving their facts to the arena.

It additionally allowed others to try and recreate their experiments to both prove or disprove their colleagues' theories.

In the case of quantum physics, the world erupted and advanced so quick inside the path of the late 19th and early twentieth centuries that it wasn't lengthy in advance than truly simply absolutely everyone worried inside the technology grow to be each constructing upon, enhancing, or downright disproving all people else's theories. One of the subjects that has stood the check of time, however, is de Broglie's speculation and de Broglie's equation. It did have a hiccup, even though, while the model of the atom shifted from the Bohr version to the more correct and superior version proposed via using Erwin Schrödinger in 1926.

Rethinking Atomic Structure and Particle-Wave Duality

Through the art work of Planck, Einstein, and de Broglie, theories approximately the real nature of particles had been being created, tested, and tailored to new studies at an awesome charge at a few degree inside the primary few a long term of the 1900s. At the equal time, distinct physicists persisted to refine and recreate the strolling model of the atom.

While those branches of research have been happening independently, the effect and intertwining of this artwork are simple. When Planck and Einstein were embroiled their work on photon idea and particle-wave duality, the Bohr version of the atom emerge as the simplest that turn out to be normally general.

As de Broglie worked to growth and show his speculation to increase particle-wave duality to encompass electrons and unique subatomic particles, Schrödinger launched his up to date version of the atom.

While the Rutherford and Bohr fashions were, and live, fantastic examples for education the essential structure of an atom, the Schrödinger version is a extra accurate depiction of the behavior of the subatomic debris. This model isn't the 2-dimensional photograph we consider while we imagine the models we first discovered approximately in university.

The Schrödinger version is a 3-dimensional view of the atom that gives scientists a extra specific concept of what the electrons of an atom are doing at any given time and additionally gave upward push to Schrödinger's equation.

This mathematical sentence is what gave the Austrian physicist the nickname "the father of quantum mechanics".

Before we get earlier of ourselves, allow's make the connection among Schrödinger's equation, the

de Broglie hypothesis, and their combined impact on the arena of quantum physics. Schrödinger's equation, that is written as:

$E\psi = H\psi$

and may be very similar in characteristic to de Broglie's equation,

$\lambda = h/mv$.

Because this is quantum physics for beginners, and Schrödinger's equation is NOT for novices, we've used the great form right right here and will supply it the most number one definition.

The most important takeaway we want you to have been the connection that this equation has with the de Broglie equation and the way they art work collectively to form the idea of quantum mechanics and quantum physics.

Schrödinger's equation is used as a predictor.

The left facet of the equation suggests the to be had strength (E) in a closed wave device and the wave characteristic (represented with the resource of the Greek letter Psi).

This indicates a prediction of wherein a particle may be at any given time in its wave motion.

It is proven inside the equation as being same to the identical wave feature and the Hamiltonian operator (H), some of that suggests the entire of the capability and kinetic strength in the device.

It appears as if every aspects of the equation are identical due to the truth they've just stated the equal problem in special methods, but that's no longer precisely the case.

Remember that the wave feature itself (the variable indicated via Psi) is the stop result of a complicated by-product equation.

Its presence on this simplified linear equation is best as it's already been calculated and canceled out.

Schrödinger superior this equation due to the fact he wanted an less complicated way to impart the capability of a particle to move alongside a wavelength. He furthermore desired to reveal that he can also want to are watching for wherein a particle may be at any given time. Remember, Schrödinger is likewise recounted for his well-known concept on a cat in a closed devicein which he posited that a cat in a field ought to probably be dead or alive and had an same hazard of being in kingdom.

Still, no person must make certain till the field became opened, and the cat turn out to be placed. It have grow to be this form of philosophy that the eccentric scientist injected into his wave prediction equation. Schrödinger desired so that you can discover a manner to convert the opportunity that a particle might be in a selected area proper right into a linear equation that would constitute that behavior.

If you are uncertain of any part of the equation, you could, much like Avogadro's equation that we mentioned in Chapter 1, plug in any of the variables to determine the numbers you are lacking.

Relating Schrödinger's Equation to de Broglie's Equation

Schrödinger's equation can be complex, however de Broglie's, fortunately, isn't. When the first equation become published in 1924, de Broglie took a take a look at it and concept it turn out to be splendid, however he needed something much less tough so as to carry out his experiments and calculate the numbers which have been going to help him in his research. Schrödinger's equation helped de Broglie gain a higher expertise of wave function, in the long run main to being able to bring together his equation for wavelength. Here's the element, despite the fact that. De Broglie has a second, lesser-recognized equation, and when you take a look at that second equation, it all starts offevolved to come back together.

$$\lambda = h/mv$$

To recap, Schrödinger's equation suggests us the predictability of wave feature, and de Broglie's equation indicates us a manner to calculate wavelength based totally totally on the momentum (mass times pace) of a particle. So, what does de Broglie's 2nd equation inform us, and how does it further relate to this early take a look at of quantum mechanics?

de Broglie's 2nd equation is written as follows:

$f = E/h$

This equation shows that the frequency (f) of a particle wave is equal to its power (E) divided by using the usage of Planck's Constant (h). You probably experience like we're strolling backward because of the truth that we haven't talked about the origins of Planck's Constant but, however we are capable of. It may be lots less difficult to recognize its entire this means that and effect in case you first recognize what a huge function it plays within the equations which might be maximum applied in quantum physics and quantum mechanics. So, with smooth equations derived from Schrödinger's complex equation, de Broglie is able to offer an cause of every the conduct of wavelength through the years and the frequency of waves given their energy degrees. Fantastic! So how did the evolution of the version of the atom from the linear, -dimensional Bohr version to the greater superior version, proposed by means of the usage of Schrödinger himself, have an effect at the manner that physicists dealt with duality and wave feature going ahead?

Adapting the Fundamentals as Knowledge Evolved

Up till 1926, maximum physicists advanced and executed their experiments the use of the Bohr model of the atom, which, as you'll recall, confirmed electrons visiting in regular orbits across the nucleus.

Once Erwin Schrödinger proposed his equation for predicting in which electrons can be based totally on their capability motion, Louis de Broglie have become able to follow up along along together with his equation to decide the wavelength of debris. It quick have come to be obvious that electrons have been probable no longer following the neat, spherical routes depicted in Bohr's model.

Schrödinger proposed a brand new running model of the atom in 1926, and it fast have emerge as substantially regular due to the fact the "quantum mechanical version."

This model is still in use these days. The reason this model is extra accurate is that the Bohr version is more often than not - dimensional. It is prepared in so-known as valence shells, with the electrons more likely to be excited and peel off traveling inside the outer orbits, and the greater stable electrons are hooked up as visiting toward the nucleus. The Bohr model remains a first-rate model for teaching the fundamentals of atomic chemistry and physics to younger university students, but the physicists who labored and keep to paintings to develop the know-how of quantum behavior wanted a few factor within the direction of a real, three-dimensional jogging version of the atom. Enter Schrödinger's model.

Schrödinger recognized that the electrons are not pleasant in constant motion but are behaving as waves in place of as particles. His model, the quantum mechanical version, presentations that evolution in information particle behavior. Schrödinger felt that his model ought to more as it ought to be represent the constant fluctuation that occurs within an electron's orbit as it's miles driven and pulled via the use of the gravitational pressure of the nucleus. Rather than surely the electrons inside the outer valence shell of Bohr's model, any electron that befell to be close to the outer type of the gravitational location would be the ones most probably to slough off or shape connections with super atoms to make molecules.

Today, scientists use the quantum mechanical model of the atom as a foundation for their experimentation.

They will regularly additionally use the time period "opportunity cloud" to explain what they see in terms of the region of an atom's electrons. The exquisite benefit of the Schrödinger model is that it is based mostly on mathematical equations that can be calculated to expose what an atom need to be doing, regardless of the truth that the motion cannot be decided. The drawback to this version is that although a scientist has the capability to study atomic behavior, wave movement on the particle level continues to be almost imperceptible. Even even though researchers understand this model to be mathematically sound, they will nevertheless lack the capability to have a observe it in movement and display it to be right. This is why some scientists are worried that this version doesn't satisfy the Heisenberg uncertainty precept, at the same time as others preserve that it does.

We'll be discussing that maximum vital later in the e-book, so you can keep in mind the evidence and decide for your self. For now, allow's pass without delay to records, definition, and realistic programs of the range you've been looking forward to, Planck's Constant.

Chapter 4: The Planck Constant

We've already stated the Planck Constant or Planck's Constant in several contexts within the first few chapters of this e-book. It elements into many equations which might be used often within the quantum physics community, so it's time to take a near test its writer Max Planck, and why his art work modified into so crucial to the improvement of the understanding of particle-wave duality.

Max Planck and His Early Work

Max Planck have become a German physicist who came from a big family of college students and academics. He received an awful lot of his grade-school diploma schooling in Munich, in which he excelled in mathematics and mechanics, and changed into moreover acknowledged to be musically proficient, education to sing and play a couple of devices. By all debts, he ought to have pursued a career in classical normal overall performance but as an opportunity decided on to conform along with his dream of being a physicist. By the early Eighteen Eighties, Planck changed into considered to be one of the brightest growing more youthful stars within the place, and thru the end of that decade, he had already climbed his way up the ladder of academia to take a publish at the Friedrich-Wilhelms-Universität in Berlin. When he retired from this position in 1926, he have grow to be succeeded with the resource of none other than Erwin Schrödinger.

Planck modified into curious about thermodynamics, and hundreds of his early research, along with that for his first doctoral diploma, targeted in this look at. He have become also interested by entropy, a idea which he felt "spooked" hundreds of his colleagues.

His papers provided the idea for loads others to begin proving their very own theories, in conjunction with that of Svante Arrhenius's hypothesis of electrolytic dissolution. Planck can also come to be a miles well-known lecturer, packing halls of fascinated college students, lots of whom praised him due to the fact the first rate speaker they'd ever heard.

Planck's many professional accomplishments, together with prevailing the 1918 Nobel Prize for Physics for his discovery of power quanta, had been finished over the direction of an entire life of personal loss.

War described most of the moments of the physicist's lifestyles, beginning with the Prussian conflicts as a little one and culminating inside the tragic loss of loads of his non-public papers and research within the path of the bombing of Berlin in WWII. He out of region a son on the Battle of Verdun in WWI, another son have come to be hanged as a traitor by way of the Nazis in 1945, and each his daughters died in childbirth.

He changed into widowed whilst he out of vicinity his first spouse Marie to tuberculosis in 1918. He remarried and become survived thru simplest his youngest little one, a son named Hermann, and his 2nd wife, Marga.

During the ones times of personal and expert turmoil, Planck remained ever the stoic German, refusing to expose his decrease again on his Jewish colleagues throughout the rise of the Third Reich and in some unspecified time in the future of World War II. As the top of Germany's maximum distinguished medical societies, he located the motto of "persevere and hold going for walks" and recommended his contemporaries to do the identical. He should keep to lecture until he neared his loss of lifestyles in 1947, but his legacy within the place of quantum physics keeps to in recent times.

Black Bodies and the Electromagnetic Spectrum

Planck's paintings and the improvement of the regular stemmed from his research into the electromagnetic spectrum and his principle at the conduct of black our our our bodies. A black body is rely which collects and absorbs every particle of radiation with which it comes in touch. Furthermore, Planck hypothesized that the frame could not best take in all that radiation, but it could, in turn, hold it and re-radiate it later.

Think of getting a white cat and a couple of black pants.

If the cat sleeps on those pants, they'll enchantment to and preserve onto maximum, if not all, of the fur that the cat sheds onto them. When you shake the pants, what takes place?

The fur starts offevolved to fly again from the cloth and into the encircling surroundings. Planck desired to apprehend if a black frame, in a vacuum, must accumulate, absorb, after which radiate all the strength it encountered, or if it had to be acted upon by means of manner of an outdoor pressure for this to rise up. He modified into furthermore curious to recognize what could seem in an open system, along with the cat and the pants. Black-body radiation relies upon upon thermodynamics and thermostability.

For this reason, it is also every so often known as thermal radiation or temperature radiation.

On a huge scale, the amazing instance of black-frame radiation is a black hollow, which absorbs everything internal a radius commensurate with its mass.

As it absorbs greater mass and strength, it starts offevolved offevolved offevolved to expand and boom its radius or "occasion horizon", growing its gravitational pull. Because it absorbs all electromagnetic waves, along with the seen slight spectrum, the "hollow" seems black.

Remember, a black hollow isn't a literal hole, however an item that's mass is so dense, it appears as a colorless singularity. Planck, and plenty of others, theorized that a black hollow maintains the strength and mass that it collects, however that, like numerous topics, might gain a breaking factor and start radiating all that power lower back outward.

He hypothesized that any alternate in temperature or big energy fluctuation would possibly throw off the device the black body modified into going for walks in and pressure reversal of the absorption; in extraordinary terms, the black frame will start radiating all the power that it formerly took in. Much later, famed physicist Dr. Stephen Hawking could hypothesize that black holes and black our bodies are continuously re-radiating absorbed energy, based totally on thermodynamic adjustments discovered along the event horizons of acknowledged black holes. There are, of course, moreover theoretical physicists who receive as proper with that singularities which includes black holes may be the crucial factor to time journey, but we'll communicate approximately that a hint bit in our bankruptcy on Einstein.

Planck's Law and Development of the Constant

So, you will be questioning what black holes, which is probably huge, want to do with quantum physics, which offers with microscopic particles. Planck become targeted on locating an cause for the behavior of seen slight and the temperature at which radiation absorbed thru and radiation emitted through a black body accumulate equilibrium. For example, the solar can be taken into consideration a black body, no matter the fact that imperfect, because it each includes enough mass to gravitationally entice radiation from the area spherical it and emit radiation decrease once more within the shape of slight and heat. The temperature at which the sun reaches equilibrium is five,777 levels Kelvin (9938° F, 5503°C). This range is likewise called the "powerful temperature". The powerful temperature varies thru the black body.

Planck were attempting to find a manner to work thru a problem known as the "Ultraviolet Catastrophe", which we're capable of all agree is a as a substitute dramatic call for a physics conundrum.

The ultraviolet catastrophe changed into an anomaly being observed by the usage of physicists trying to provide an motive for the behavior of black our our bodies as they emitted radiation.

Many of Planck's contemporaries were looking this catastrophic occasion of their studies.

While the scientists believed that a black-body need to radiate power at a regular charge within the route of the huge electromagnetic spectrum, they have been as an alternative locating that the black-our our bodies were emitting big portions of radiation in high-electricity, immoderate-frequency bursts, which may also all at once burn up the absorbed power and drop the gadget proper down to internet-0 quicker than predicted. This effect become most usually determined due to the truth the strength being radiated reached the ultraviolet form of the electromagnetic spectrum.

In his tries to understand and solve the ultraviolet catastrophe, Planck placed that the trouble with the classical physics being finished to the conundrum became that they didn't account for the entire spectrum of electromagnetic radiation to drop in frequency and wavelength over the years and alternate in temperature.

By which incorporates those variables into the equation, Planck turn out to be capable of boom Planck's Law.

It makes use of arithmetic to explain the connection most of the energy absorbed thru a black-body and the price of launch of that radiation at a high quality temperature, considering that the rate of energy exchange can also want to exceptional be emitted in increments proportional to the spectral density of the electromagnetic wave.

In simplified terms, Planck's Law describes a closed machine wherein the electricity absorbed, and the electricity radiated via manner of using a black-body beneath a ordinary temperature live in equilibrium however money owed for adjustments in frequency and wavelength of the radiation given the potential strength and internet-zero nature of the closed device.

When carried out arithmetic is used to expose Planck's Law, the outcomes may be plotted on a curve that suggests that the frequency of the electromagnetic waves will fall off after a certain time, given the shape of radiation. Planck and his colleagues mentioned this motion as spectral density. The capability to unique this conduct drastically advanced the arena of quantum physics and separated it even in addition from classical theorists.

Many scientists mark the book of Planck's Law in 1901 as the "starting" of modern quantum physics.

Measurement and conduct Planck's regular in motion

One of the critical thing elements in developing Planck's Law is the use of the amount we're all proper right here for, Planck's Constant. The consistent is referenced in Planck's previous artwork but wouldn't be universally identified as a mathematical regular till after 1905. There's a sincere way to keep in mind Planck's Constant, even earlier than we get into any math. The foundation in the returned of the constant end up Planck's preference to place a call or unit to the smallest viable quantity of electricity. That's all. Planck knew that the smallest pieces of be counted were determined (at the time, this have end up the atom and its subatomic factors). He favored a way to "quantize" or degree power at its tiniest little wave. It become in his pursuit of this that Planck's Constant modified into born. Behold, the mathematical object of our affection:

h =6.6262 x 10-34 Joule •second

Let's ruin down what the numbers imply and how Planck got here to them.

Frankly, the h is virtually the variable letter that Planck selected because it wasn't getting used to represent something else in mathematics or the budding field of quantum physics.

The SI unit joule-2nd isn't always to be careworn with joules consistent with 2d. A joule-second stands on my own as a unit to degree on every occasion and movement.

Now for the huge variety itself. 6.6262 x 10-34 is a sincerely tiny amount that represents the quantity of power that is produced by the usage of a unmarried particle. We recognize that all debris vibrate.

Planck modified into the first to quantify or "quantize" that vibration.

The only manner that Planck's Constant is used is to determine the strength of a photon via multiplying the normal through the photon's frequency. This works because of the reality we recognize that a particle's, together with a photon's, mass is equal to its power. No rely which variables you personal, you may be able to calculate those you are missing, and all because of Planck's Constant. For example:

$E = h f$

In this favored equation showing using Planck's Constant, we see that the strength (E) of a photon or particle is same to the frequency (f) times the constant. This equation become superior as part of the Planck-Einstein relation and is a critical precept of quantum physics and quantum mechanics.

It emerge as this equation that de Broglie took on step similarly in growing his very very own, which, as we understand, calculates the conduct of a wave based totally totally on its momentum. Planck's Constant furthermore plays carefully into the Heisenberg

Uncertainty Principle, which we'll explore in some intensity in the next chapter.

Development and use of Planck's decreased Constant every different use for Planck

Another use for Planck's Constant is in its decreased form, symbolized via way of the usage of the h-bar, which seems like this: ℏ. The h-bar is implemented in vicinity of the equal vintage h in calculations which might be factoring in angular momentum in desire to linear momentum. Linear momentum is, of route, calculated thru multiplying mass times velocity.

It depicts the momentum of an item or particle as it travels along planes, most often in a right now line. Angular momentum is a made from calculating momentum in 3 dimensions.

A commonplace example of this will be a gyroscope, which has the functionality of shifting in numerous hints and keeps its movement via the capability to alter to those dimensions.

In classical physics, angular momentum is calculated through the sum of the momentum of all the moving factors, but this doesn't normally paintings on a quantum scale. In order for physicists in case you want to as it must be determine the momentum of particles in 3 dimensions on a quantum scale, a brand new equation modified into desired. By using the Planck Constant in its general shape, physicists can use the de Broglie equation to treatment for unknown momentums. For solving for unknown momentums within the case of a particle showing angular momentum, a derivative of the Planck Constant grow to be created, which we now name Planck's Reduced Constant, and the ħ represents this new charge. It is decided in equation shape like so:

$$\hbar = h$$

$$2\pi$$

As you could see, the Planck Constant divided with the resource of instances pi gives us the reduced Planck Constant.

Why does this art work to find out unknown variables in problems associated with particles transferring in three dimensions?

To apprehend this, you need to additionally recognize that a wave is part of a parabola.

We apprehend that if a parabola is extrapolated past its curve, it can in the end be a part of and shape a whole circle or 360°.

However, waves don't certainly flip another time on themselves and complete a 360° circle.

Instead, scientists degree one complete wave cycle, from its beginning aircraft (the baseline) as masses because the pinnacle of its amplitude (the crest) and backtrack thru the baseline to its lowest aspect (the trough) as 360°.

Each time the wave completes this motion is measured as one hertz, and that is taken into consideration the frequency of the wave.

This is not to be confused with wavelength, which measures the distance among the crests of a wave.

By dividing the Planck Constant via 2π (the usual equation for identifying the circumference of a 360* circle or wave frequency), the decreased regular can be used to calculate the momentum of items or particles which is probably moving along a couple of plane at a time. An example of adapting de Broglie's equation to apply the reduced Planck Constant is:

$p = \hbar$ good enough

In this situation, the variable p stands for momentum, the h-bar suggests Planck's Reduced Constant (calculated with the useful resource of manner of the usage of the frequency of the wave in question), and the ok represents the angular wavenumber.

Angular wavenumber is an overstated time period for the size of waves taking place over a tremendous distance, in place of measuring them in time.

While Planck's Reduced Constant isn't used nearly as heaps as the same old constant, it is useful in determining the movement and momentum in the ones instances wherein a particle or object is visiting along greater than planes.

Planck himself turned into often nonchalant approximately his work and might regularly tell humans, as within the case of the everyday, that he changed into truely seeking out numbers that could make one of a kind numbers make revel in.

He even once noted the regular as a "math trick." He was a excellent mind who likely discounted most of his very personal studies to an surrender, and Planck could probable be amazed approximately the impact of his legacy in the future development of quantum physics. But fact be suggested, without

Planck, his prison tips, and his steady, man can also have in no way finished area tour or built advanced studies machine on the side of the Large Hadron Collider.

Chapter 5: Heisenberg's Uncertainty Principle

We've all been uncertain at times.

Do we want the chicken or the fish? Which movie are we able to want to look?

Eventually, you make a decision, and the uncertainty is lengthy beyond. But to recognize the subsequent idea we're about to address, you want to remember being both certain, and unsure on the equal time. Heisenberg's Uncertainty Principle, which he brought to the area in 1927, dreams to provide an cause of certainly one of quantum mechanics' largest troubles, how can one count on in which a particle might be at any given time, irrespective of the records of its momentum or preceding position? First, permit's test Heisenberg's paintings that led him as a good deal because the Uncertainty Principle.

Heisenberg's Beginnings in Physics

Werner Heisenberg modified into born in Germany to educational parents. His father emerge as a professor of ancient languages and Greek philosophy, and more youthful Werner loved to interact in philosophical discussions with his non-public teachers and pals. He spoke nearly lovingly of the atom as a philosophical pursuit, which can only be reliably accounted for with mathematics.

He might also test beneath and with a number of the alternative super scientific minds of his time, collectively with Niels Bohr himself.

Heisenberg modified into moreover musically gifted, a common thread amongst a number of the pioneering physicists.

His propensity for the piano led him to satisfy his future spouse, Elizabeth, after a normal overall performance. She changed into additionally from an academic own family and endorsed him at some point of his career to push his theories and studies to new heights of discovery. The physicist was furthermore an avid outdoorsman, lively in many jobs with the German Scouts all through his lifetime.

He might regularly retreat to the mountains while he became thinking thru a honestly hard physics or mathematical trouble.

While he's in particular acknowledged nowadays for his well-known uncertainty precept, Heisenberg's earliest predominant art work turn out to be a collaboration borne from his doctoral thesis.

In partnership with Max Born and Pascual Jordan, Heisenberg proposed a hard and fast of mathematical matrices that might be used to provide an reason for and anticipate the movement of atomic particles with reference to mechanical strategies. Unfortunately for Heisenberg and his colleagues, they have been in the Bohr camp of theoretical physics, which have become slowly being phased out for the more present day paintings of Einstein, Planck, Schrödinger, de Broglie. While classical physics and mathematics had been however a basis of the greater moderen fields of quantum physics, quantum mechanics, and atomic research, the disciplines were experiencing a unexpectedly widening hollow in beliefs and thoughts. While Heisenberg's mechanical matrices have been no longer universally regularly occurring or utilized by the physics network, they weren't with out benefit.

Part of the cause they fell through way of the wayside is that Bohr's university became falling out of style as being vintage.

While this appears a chunk ridiculous given the velocity at which new quantum discoveries had been being made, Bohr and his contemporaries and university college students were firmly entrenched inside the physical houses of the atom as a real, tangible item.

While the Einstein camp became analyzing wave-particle duality, the Bohr camp grow to be concerned with what they known as discrete bundlesquantum particles traveling together in packets of power. They weren't interested in some thing they couldn't degree via commentary or assume with 100% fact.

While Heisenberg ought to circulate far from his previous colleagues in idea and motion, due in part to Jordan leaving academia to end up as Nazi SS officer within the Thirties, he might in all likelihood, later in life, deliver credit score to Born and Jordan as being instrumental to his early improvement and eventual reception of the Nobel Prize.

Heisenberg himself would possibly spend masses of the 1930s and Nineteen Forties beneath the scrutiny of the Nazis.

They deemed his artwork to be counterproductive to their hobby in harnessing nuclear electricity truly for the reason of weaponization.

The Development of the Uncertainty Principle

The Heisenberg Uncertainty Principle has emerge as Heisenberg's lasting legacy inside the worldwide of particle physics, and it end up a long time in improvement and refinement. Heisenberg ought to in no way honestly depart inside the once more of his belief within the Bohr school of test. Still, he ought to ultimately need to apprehend that the artwork of those inside the Einstein university modified into garnering more interest. Heisenberg's views of the studies completed through humans who have been working alongside facet Einstein have been complex. He saw their paintings as dealing in "reality" and taken into attention himself an "antirealist". The contradiction proper proper right here is that Heisenberg cherished the mathematics of physics, which deals generally in reality. Numbers are absolutes and are very real.

So, wherein did the Uncertainty Principle stem from?

Let's take a look at the fundamental premise of the Uncertainty Principle (which, with the resource of the manner, Heisenberg himself, known as the Indeterminacy Principle).

It states that it's miles impossible to recognize every the vicinity and the momentum of a particle at the equal time, even the use of commentary, predictors, and equations.

That's a quite, bold assertion, so permit's test why it's far each real and arguable. Obviously, if you can see and diploma some detail, then definitely it is precisely what you suspect it is and in which you assume it to be.

To in the interim, scientists argue this factor. Many enjoy that the measuring of debris with precision is the handiest manner to make certain in their behavior.

Why should Heisenberg be so unsure approximately this?

Heisenberg postulated that the person of quantum motion is that there is a limit to how masses facts viable benefit from it. He believed that there were forces at paintings inner a quantum system that had been beyond the scope of human commentary and knowledge. Heisenberg went to this point as to theorize that the greater as it have to be one variable inside a machine can be measured, the extra the inaccuracy of each other duration. In easy phrases, the extra precise the dimensions of the placement of a particle, the lots plenty less particular the scale of its momentum, and vice versa.

Why might in all likelihood he anticipate this?

And greater to the component, have to he show it together collectively together with his preferred mathematics?

Using his formerly provided mechanical matrices, Heisenberg set out to reveal his indeterminacy principle, and terrific sufficient, given the tiniest versions in particle motion and momentum, he proceeded to expose that a, times b, didn't typically identical b time a.

The infinitesimal variations he decided in quantum movement served due to the truth the mathematical basis for what would possibly turn out to be the Uncertainty Principle.

Remember, Heisenberg and his colleagues were concerned greater often than no longer with mechanical systems, because of this that the particles were not present in a vacuum, as with electromagnetic structures. Heisenberg concluded that the existence of even the most minuscule out of doors forces had been causing the atoms to act in a way that made statement and dimension limited in scope, thereby limiting the know-how one must advantage from studying the tool.

Because he have come to be furthermore a person of philosophy and movement, Heisenberg moreover finished what his cohorts deemed a "concept check", regardless of the truth that Niels Bohr may additionally later admit that the scientific foundation of the studies became sound. To perform this take a look at, Heisenberg attempted to study the conduct of atomic debris, especially electrons, using a gamma-ray microscope.

While watching those debris, he determined that the gamma radiation become appearing in the direction of the herbal movement of the debris.

It have become basically "kicking" the electrons round, now not permitting him to get an accurate picture of what the particle must be doing in their natural usa of the us. To get a greater unique reading at the conduct of the electrons, Heisenberg then performed a stronger, more correct microscope to the particles.

What passed off changed into even more unpredictability from the electrons, which have been now being acted upon via energy from the stronger microscope.

Heisenberg in the long run posited that it turned into a hassle of the man or woman of quantum movement itself and no longer the scope or boundaries of the observational device itself that created the uncertainty paradox.

Every time he completed an commentary tool that emitted greater energy, he injected that energy into the device and similarly advanced the uncertainty. In the most easy of terms, it isn't always possible to realise what a particle will do, even in case you recognise wherein it's far.

If you understand what it's miles doing, you can't pinpoint its actual region. This principle is now one of the foundations of particle physics, quantum mechanics, quantum chemistry, and theoretical physics.

When scientists need to use Heisenberg's Uncertainty Principle in their paintings, they test all the mitigating elements that would have an impact on their measurements and observations, together with the skills and obstacles in their laboratory system.

They additionally recollect the accuracy of their baseline information, the self perception they have got in their preceding or preparatory paintings and the art work of others, and the previously seemed uncertainty of similar experiments or substances.

By amassing and collating this records before starting an test, physicists and chemists can decide the functionality for variations and margins of errors inside their research.

Mathematics uncertainty and the Planck Constant in Action

When developing an equation to explicit the Uncertainty Principle in actionable phrases, it end up essential for Heisenberg to lease Planck's Reduced Constant, or the h-bar, that we referred to within the remaining financial break. The simplest shape of this equation is installed right here:

This equation is a visible illustration of the precept, and you may see Planck's Reduced Constant at the right issue of the mathematical sentence.

It is split via because of the truth there are variables at the left aspect of the equation.

On that left issue, we see Greek deltas, which might be the uncertainties.

The Δ placed via the variable x represents the size of the location of a quantum particle, and the Δ discovered through the variable px, which represents the dimensions of the particle's momentum.

The Δ itself stands for the same old deviation.

When we positioned it all collectively, the entire equation reads, "The massive deviation of the location times the identical antique deviation of the momentum is greater than or same to 1/2 of of Planck's Reduced Constant."

Broken down like this, it's now not hard to appearance what Heisenberg become getting at alongside together together with his precept.

The modern day deviation is the amount above or under a predicted or previously measured region wherein the particle may be predicted to be placed or its anticipated or previously measured momentum.

This will range with the beneficial resource of particle and condition, of course.

He predicted that those quantities expanded with the useful resource of each distinctive would possibly constantly pop out to an equal or huge variety than the reduced normal divided with the beneficial useful resource of the style of variables. If the wide variety have been ever to pop out much less, that could imply that the placement and momentum of the debris have been anticipated with one hundred percent accuracy earlier than they even came into the arena of operation, this is statistically quite, pretty improbable.

Separating uncertainty from the observer effect

Within all of generation, there may be a puzzle known as the Observer Effect. The premise of this impact is easy; on every occasion an observation is made through each human, mechanical, or virtual manner, the results of the statement are affected by the very act.

So, does that propose that each one research results are faux?

No, and the model in results is so typically so minimal that they're nearly undetectable.

However, those versions nonetheless exist.

They aren't, no matter the truth that, to be stressed with the Uncertainty Principle.

The Uncertainty Principle want to be held in separate regard as the Observer Effect due to the reality the Observer Effect is found in almost every trouble of life, on each a microscopic and macroscopic scale.

You cannot see in a dark room with out acting upon it with a slight supply. You can't have a look at an atomic particle with out a few tool with which to perform your observations. Each time we strive to take a look at some thing, we want to act upon it with a few outside pressure, an amazing manner to then enact exchange on the gadget. There additionally seems to three misinformation or misconceptions that the observer is always human, and that human mistakes or interference is the defining factor within the Observer Effect.

This isn't real, the Observer Effect additionally occurs in the case of mechanical, robot, or virtual observational tools. The problem is that it's far not possible to behavior any research with out research system.

We'd never have the capacity to research a few detail!

Thankfully, the real results of remark are especially innocent and can be calculated away with a margin of mistakes. This is, of course, barring any clearly catastrophic interaction, together with knocking over a whole check or a few one in every of a kind freak incidence.

Corrections, rebuttals, and variations of the Uncertainty Principle

A lot has happened inside the medical global thinking about the truth that Heisenberg first introduced the Uncertainty Principle, and over the numerous years, it's had its honest proportion of controversy and variations.

There is a camp, albeit small of cutting-edge scientists who've refuted the Heisenberg Uncertainty Principle in its entirety.

There is also a larger contingent who feels that the precept's spirit need to be upheld but that it needs a few changes or clarifications to live suitable for use.

Since the Uncertainty Principle can only be finished to quantum-degree have a observe, many scientists enjoy the want to conform it as plenty as a macro degree, however that's no longer mathematically viable. The precept best applies to quantum fabric because of the reality classical physics has the method to proper now take a look at the region and momentum of devices without the use of tool so that you can have an effect on the variables. In quantum mechanics, it is important to use period and commentary tools as a manner to impact the device. This is one of the essential versions among classical and quantum physics and mechanics.

There is likewise a university of idea that really dismisses the Uncertainty Principle and truely embraces Schrödinger's wave equation, no matter the fact that this isn't the fairest approach both, due to the fact quantum physics and quantum mechanics deal with sides of the identical coin of atomic predictability and measurability.

The Uncertainty Principle gives extra flexibility inside the interpretation of records, that is ironic given Heisenberg's devotion to the absolutes of arithmetic however not surprising, given his equal love of philosophy and rhetoric.

No rely which college of perception you fall into, the Uncertainty Principle come to be and will stay a landmark within the improvement of particle physics and quantum mechanics. There are many who reject it totally because of the truth they don't want to consider the opportunity of being now not able to recognize everything approximately particle behavior regardless of the truth that we've got were given were given the gadget to check and diploma it.

While the arena is populated with many brave humans, fear of the unknown is a restricting behavior of people and isn't probable to be overcome any time fast.

The final debatable concept we'll provide about the Uncertainty Principle is this, and it's in useful resource of the rule of thumb: if instrumentation has grow to be more and more particular through the years, why does the precept nevertheless maintain?

There are many that trust it's best end up extra prescient, as modern-day instrumentation is stronger and greater accurate than it has ever been.

It's as loads as you to decide the manner you revel in about the Uncertainty Principle, however probably you could take an prolonged hike in the mountains and consider it, a bargain as Heisenberg himself may have.

Chapter 6: Einstein And His Foundational Physics

We've come to our very last financial disaster, and yes, we stored the maximum important call (and face) in quantum physics for the grand finale. Albert Einstein emerge as no longer exceptional one of era's most remarkable members, however he turned into moreover one of the most prolific. Einstein is understood across the world for being a pioneer inside the observe and understanding of quantum physics. Let's take a detailed have a take a look at the person himself and some of his most important, lasting accomplishments and contributions to the sector of physics.

Early Life and Work

Albert Einstein became born inside the Kingdom of Württemberg, a country of the German Empire, in 1879. Although his family come to be non-training Jewish, he might attend a Catholic school for his early early life schooling. He spent a variety of that youth in

Munich, in which his father and uncle constructed and ran an electrical deliver business enterprise. Einstein excelled in math and technological information, writing wonderful papers on count number states in advance than the age of sixteen. At the encouragement of his uncle, he started teaching himself Euclidean geometry and algebra and reading track and philosophy in his early teenagers. Young Albert passed every teach his own family ought to offer for him and come to be admitted to university on the Swiss Federal Technical School on his second strive at the doorway assessments. He'd failed the number one because of a lack of elegant training.

With his father's permission, Einstein renounced his German citizenship and characteristic become a Swiss citizen to keep away from compulsory military issuer. He may additionally graduate from the technical school with top marks however can be frustrated at the shortage of coaching positions in his location. Unable to find an educational method, the ought to-be scientist took a process in Switzerland's federal patent place of worka preference that can exchange the route of technology history.

While running on the patent administrative center, Einstein reviewed some of programs for improvements that claimed to harness electric powered alerts.

It become those patent applications that could jumpstart Einstein's fascination with the connection between charged debris and the character of touring atoms and slight.

Not content material material to waste away in a low-degree authorities method, Einstein worked inside the course of his superior levels and noted technological understanding and philosophy along along together with his pals. He have become subsequently furnished his doctorate from the University of Zurich in 1905, kicking off what has been referred to as his "miracle three hundred and sixty five days", and to be frank, what he completed in

1905 on my own is going to soak up most of the rest of the financial ruin.

Not first-rate did he gift and shield his thesis at the willpower of molecular dimensions, however he moreover published essential papers on Brownian motion, the photoelectric effect, the principle of particular relativity, and the mass equivalency equation, that is now known as the maximum famous equation inside the international. It have to be noted; this became the three hundred and sixty five days that Einstein grew to turn out to be actually 26 years antique.

Brownian Motion

Einstein's first leap forward paper of 1905 became his treatise on Brownian motion. In the best of terms, Brownian movement is the random motion of particles on the same time as suspended in a gasoline or fluid. This phenomenon is so-called for a botanist named Robert Brown who, in 1827, observed the motion of pollen suspended in water. Einstein come to be the first to lend any immoderate credence to Brown's notes of the occasion.

When Einstein published his paper, he did so you can lend his guide that Brownian motion changed into the cease end result of the presence of atoms and molecules within the water, offering a conduit for the debris of pollen to transport. Because the strength of everyone molecule technique that there may be no steady to the stress being positioned upon the suspended particles, their motion is found as being random.

Taking this precept, a touch bit in addition is the concept that now not one of the bombarded and bounced-approximately particles may be counted due to their randomness, nor can the atoms or molecules that make up the active medium. However, Einstein did create equations to accompany his theories, irrespective of the truth that every equations (each approximately a web page lengthy) have been changed with simplified versions created through special scientists.

Despite his equations being phased out, and no matter the theory of Brownian movement being confirmed in 1909 by means of manner of Jean Perrin, in region of through Einstein himself, the genuine credit rating for the concept stays with Einstein.

In authentic Einstein style, he became more amused with the resource of the initial snub of his principle than he changed into pleased with it whilst it modified into subsequently demonstrated.

Einstein's tackle Brownian motion could probably show instrumental within the development of numerous other theories with the useful resource of both classical and theoretical physicists and those who've been getting concerned within the budding fields of quantum physics and quantum mechanics. Not the least of these subsequent theories are the kinetic principle of heat, Stoke's law, and the ideal regulation of fuel.

The Photoelectric Effect

The photoelectric effect is some specific one in all Einstein's 1905 bounce forward hypotheses, and it might trade the medical global's view on the manner moderate travels and is transmitted. The photoelectric effect have become recognized via way of using Einstein due to the fact the emission of electrons from a material while it's far hit with electromagnetic radiation within the mild spectrum. In unique phrases, whilst mild (ultraviolet via infrared) touches a substance, it causes that substance to launch electrons. The cause that Einstein's paper became so innovative is that it have become in direct contradiction to the electromagnetic precept of classical physics. That model confirmed a predictable glide of electrons along an electric powered powered powered area created by using way of the stress and electricity of the encircling modern-day.

In Einstein's model of photoelectricity, the electrons do not drift however are as an alternative flung from their determine substance in a as an opportunity violent way. Imagine you're status inside the the front of a wall made of sheetrock.

What can also need to show up if you threw a few issue on the wall? Depending at the momentum of what you threw, it might undergo the wall. It might also look off the wall and fly back at you.

Or it could hit the wall and lose all its momentum and tumble to the floor. No rely which of those three reactions takes place, one issue is positive, and this is that bits of drywall are going to be launched from the wall whilst and from wherein your item hits it.

You can reflect onconsideration on the wall because of the reality the take a look at substance, the object you throw as a beam of moderate strength, and the drywall that flies off the wall because the electrons being launched.

Einstein emerge as in truth now not the primary to signify the photoelectric impact, however he come to be the primary to be taken considerably. As early because of the truth the 1860s, scientists were suggesting that moderate had the characteristics of every particles and waves but weren't sure a way to expose it. In the past due Nineteen Eighties, Heinrich Hertz become capable of produce electromagnetic radiation. Still, he couldn't provide an explanation for why his results modified at the identical time as he used ultraviolet rays in location of visible slight or infrared. As we now understand, it's due to the fact the shorter wavelengths of ultraviolet carry greater kinetic energy and function extra momentum than the longer wavelengths of infrared radiation.

The subsequent character to deal with the mystery of mild electricity modified into JJ Thomson, who we met early on this ebook due to the fact the progenitor of the plum pudding version of the atom.

As you'll bear in thoughts, Thomson furthermore became the number one to understand electrons. It come to be a scientist named Philipp Lenard who would possibly bridge the space among Thomson and Einstein at the identical time as Lenard carried out first rate research on locating the minimal threshold at which moderate should discharge electrons from precise materials. He achieved round with increasing the intensity of his moderate sources but may also need to in no way discover an motive in the back of why the substances were behaving the manner they did. Enter Einstein, who would be the handiest to make the connections most of the conduct of moderate and its actual nature, that is that mild, having no mass, must be made from natural strength and therefore is a wave. However, as particle-wave duality tells us, moderate need to surely have a shape to tour thru place, and consequently, mild is crafted from particles which we now recognize to be photons.

Without Einstein fixing the enigma of the photoelectric impact, we would in no way have come to a entire expertise of particle wave duality.

He turn out to be able to offer an reason of why Lenard's experiments with slight intensity have been now not producing the expected resultsit wasn't the amplitude of his waves that have been missing, however as an alternative the frequency.

By increasing the frequency of the waves within the experimental technique, Einstein changed into capable of come up with the outcomes that Lenard were seeking out, which have become an increase in electrons released from a steel plate whilst hit with mild waves.

With one paper on the photoelectric impact, Einstein became the theoretical physics worldwide on its head.

By postulating that mild grow to be, in truth, a motion of debris behaving as a wave, the face of quantum physics modified all the time. In proper Einstein shape, he, of route, end up able to create a series of equations to quantify his precept, and in evaluation to his equations for Brownian movement, those ones stuck.

To placed math to paintings at the photoelectric impact, Einstein's equation seems like this:

K max = h v − W

Look! There's our vintage friend Planck's Constant, showing as lots as assist. Let's harm down what's taking area on this equation, starting with the K at the left aspect. This variable, with its subscript, stands for the most kinetic strength of the electrons at the floor earlier than being subjected to a mild wave.

On the proper facet of the equation, we see the variables we'll need to decide that most kinetic strength. The h is Planck's Constant, and it's being elevated via v, that is the frequency of the wave being carried out to the electrons. The considerable of hv then has the final variable W subtracted, W being the art work feature of the electrons. This is the minimal energy threshold had to cast off electrons from the ground.

To apprehend the paintings, function a touch bit higher, it might be useful to understand that this variable is from time to time represented as BE, which stands for binding strength.

It is the artwork of the scientist to determine what the threshold frequency is for the waves they're the usage of as opposed to the cloth they desire to get rid of electrons from. The better the frequency of the waves, the more likely the outcomes will show more electrons being launched.

This dating will boom proportionately in among substances with sturdy and robust electron bonds these materials will want electromagnetic waves of growing frequency to get them to shed their electrons.

His art work explaining the photoelectric impact changed into so seminal, it is the concept that obtained Einstein his Nobel Prize in 1921, no matter the rest of his groundbreaking theories. By categorizing light as each a wave and a particle, Einstein opened the doors for the studies and improvement of such a lot of extraordinary theories and gave shipping to a whole new worldwide of quantum opportunities.

General relativity, Special relativity, and Mass Equivalency

To understand why Einstein's theories of relativity and the idea of mass equivalency have been and live so crucial, we need to pass back in time a hint bit.

Because all of physics is constructed upon the artwork of the scientists who came earlier than, we first want to look at the two older additives that pass were the primary elements in what must grow to be Einstein's hypotheses.

The first hassle is the classical legal guidelines of motion, superior through way of way of Sir Isaac Newton inside the overdue 1600s.

From Newton's worldwide changing theories, we recognize the subsequent things:

1) A body in movement remains in movement, and a body at rest stays at relaxation except acted upon with the aid of manner of an outside pressure.

2) Force equals the trade in momentum steady with unit of change in time. In phrases of steady mass, pressure equals mass instances acceleration.

3) Every motion has an equal and opposite response.

Newton's felony pointers were the concept of classical physics and went unquestioned for nearly centuries.

It's best once they began to be examined extra carefully that the deviation between classical physics and quantum physics commenced.

Quantum particles, as we understand, do no longer behave in the equal manner macro-gadgets.

The second element we want to aspect into the background of the improvement of the theories of relativity is the invention of the speed of light and early artwork into the nature of mild.

A Scottish physicist named James Maxwell modified into the first to decide the speed of mild (186,000 miles consistent with second) in 1865, and he additionally recommended that slight well-knownshows the houses of each a wave and a particle. However, Maxwell and his colleagues remained under the have an impact on that slight required a medium via which to journey.

In the 1980s, a couple of American scientists cracked the code on whether or not or no longer slight desired a medium or if it is able to excursion in a vacuum.

It sounds similar to the beginning of a funny story, however a physicist and a chemist walked right into a bar and bet every different that they could determine out the mysteries of light.

Okay, that's now not precisely the manner it went, however the end result is that AA Michelson and Edward Morley decided that mild need no "ether" to surround it and might adventure through area and time on its very personal, thank you very a superb deal. This revelation for all time changed the manner that scientists, and anyone, keep in mind the very nature of existence.

When Einstein become handiest a youngster in the Eighteen Nineteen Nineties, he emerge as interested by the motion and nature of light, writing great papers, and acting his well-known "concept experiments" about the priority.

He would possibly write of one such take a look at, wherein he pictured himself the use of a wave of slight and noticed every other wave of slight strolling in parallel.

Despite his mass being atop the number one wave, the speed turn out to be unaffected, and the 2 beams of mild endured to excursion on the identical speed. What the more youthful Einstein has stumbled upon have become the origins of his theories of relativity.

Classical physics should have informed Einstein that if he had been atop a shifting wave, strolling in parallel to a few other wave transferring at the equal pace, then the relative pace of the waves can be internet zero.

This, but, is a right away contradiction to Maxwell's showed difficulty that mild normally travels on the equal pace, which we recognize to be 186,000 miles consistent with 2nd.

This were given Einstein to thinking, how can mild beams traveling subsequent to every specific have each the identical pace of 186,000 miles consistent with 2d however honestly have a relative pace of zero?

If you've followed along to date, proper proper here's what we are able to end: devices moving on the proper identical speed alongside the same axis could have the identical thing of view and observe the identical things.

It's all simultaneous, and their relative pace is 0. This follows the theories of classical physics, which Einstein did not disagree with However, if devices aren't transferring on the equal pace, their relative speed is the distinction the diverse speeds. Imagine trains walking on parallel tracks. One teach goes a hundred kph, and the alternative is going at 50 kph. These trains weigh the equal, leave the station concurrently, and attain their most acceleration on the identical time, however the quicker train reaches their vacation spot in half of the time due to the fact the slower educate because of the fact they have got a relative speed differential of 50 kph.

The first educate travels 100 miles over the course of 1 hour; the second one train takes two hours to gather the identical distance.

Light doesn't have this problem. Light constantly travels at the identical velocity and doesn't must worry approximately resistance, friction, or other opposing forces.

If two beams of mild modified the trains in the previous example, the ones beams of mild might in all likelihood reach their holiday spot at the identical time.

They constantly have a relative pace of zero. Now, permit's upload any other variable to this. Going lower back to trains, permit's say that a teach is journeying beyond a fixed element, like a mile marker. If there is a man status next to the mile marker even as the train passes at 100 kph, he would in all likelihood see the train traveling beyond him and will have a take a look at the whole teach. The teach and the character have a relative speed of 100 kph because of the fact the train is transferring, and the individual is desk bound.

Now, allow's positioned the individual on a teach transferring inside the opposite path on a parallel tune.

This teach is likewise shifting at 100 kph. Both trains left their locations on the identical time and performed maximum acceleration concurrently. They will skip the mile marker in the middle of the route at the same time. This mile marker will become a singularity, and now that each trains pass it, their relative speed turns into 0, and it will appear to be time has slowed down.

This is the phenomenon that Einstein have become most interested in. His hobby approximately the simultaneous nature of movement near time led right away to his introduction of the special concept of relativity and the invention of the distance-time continuum.

Einstein perplexed why, regardless of pace and feature; items want to in no way outrun mild.

He additionally confused how time played into the equation.

The precept he created approach that the speed of slight is virtually the restriction of pace inside the universe and that no item can ever overtake the price of mild due to the character of mass. Because mild has no mass, it's far the handiest problem which could journey at that tempo. He furthermore theorized that mass will increase as an object's tempo will growth and that ultimately, the item becomes so heavy that its mass will become the restricting problem. That leads us to the most famous equation inside the global, the mass equivalency equation, and it's miles brilliant in its simplicity:

E = mc2

Let's harm it down. The left aspect of the equation is in which we see the variable E, which represents the complete strength of an object. Since we recognize that mass and electricity can't be created or destroyed, we comprehend that there may be mass equivalency in gadgets that show off wave-particle duality.

This equation shows us what occurs to an item this is journeying at the squared pace of mild (notated right here with the letter c).

This is a variety of this is microscopically shy of 90,000,000,000 square kilometers constant with 2d.

This variety is then extended thru using the mass of the item, allow's say 10 kilograms. The power in that mass is now 900,000,000,000 joules.

That's a ludicrous amount of power! But it's although no longer sufficient energy to transport that object quicker than the charge of mild.

Einstein decided that the quicker an item goes, the heavier it gets. Its mass will increase, and it is physical more hard to move an object with greater mass.

As the object hurtles alongside coming near the rate of moderate, its ever-growing mass disallows it from ever attaining maximum pace. Therefore, the object will never be capable of pass quicker than the price of moderate, the quickest tempo allowable in our universe. The only declaration of the precise principle of relativity is that this: as an object approaches the charge of moderate, the within the course of countless its mass will become, because of this that it's going to by no means be able to overtake the fee of mild.

Don't fear if unique relativity seems counterintuitive to you; it felt that manner to Einstein, too, and his contemporaries.

How can some factor hold to transport that speedy and never advantage most tempo?

It's due to the reality while we think about topics shifting, we have a tendency to reflect onconsideration on them having the capability to move in 3 dimensions up and down on a vertical axis, left and right on a horizontal axis, and beforehand and backward on a rotating axis.

But Einstein located matters a bit bit in any other case and proposed that there is a fourth size that desires to be considered, and that fourth measurement is time.

Einstein posited that point MUST be accounted for whilst looking at relative motion and speeds. The concept of time because the fourth size were tossed around with the aid of way of various physicists preceding to Einstein's hobby in relativity. He saw the paintings of German mathematician Hermann Minkowski, as a brilliant foundation for running out precisely how time factored into relativity. Minkowski posted a paper in

1908 that solidified his mathematical theories on spacetime due to the fact the fourth length, and Einstein became interested about the matrices that protected time as a vector that is a constant factor, honestly due to the fact the equal vintage points alongside the x, y, and z axes may be. This have become the inspiration that led Einstein to simply accept as authentic with that point is probably used as a coordinate, and so the idea of spacetime modified into born. Einstein moreover commenced to marvel what would appear if we stopped thinking about being in motion via region and started out thinking about place transferring spherical us.

Have you ever stood on the beach and allow an ocean wave are available in over your feet and legs? You are the consistent point, and the sea is the body in movement. Yet, if you stand and stare upon a few other ordinary element on the horizon while that wave crashes over your ft, you could experience as if you are moving backward whilst the wave recedes. We sense the identical phenomenon now and again at the same time as driving alongside a multi-lane toll road. Because it isn't always statistically probably that every car is journeying at exactly the same velocity, there might be times at the same time as you observe the automobile subsequent to you and get the perception that the other vehicle is transferring backward in vicinity of you are shifting forward. These are everyday examples of relativity and the space-time continuum at artwork.

When Einstein commenced out to consider time because the fourth size, he started out to marvel why time appeared to sluggish down even as items have been accelerating.

This educate of notion is what added Einstein from the concept of unique relativity, which only involved devices journeying alongside a hard and fast aircraft at a hard and fast tempo, to the idea of modern relativity, which problems all devices in location and time shifting at quite a few speeds.

By including acceleration and time as a dimension into his issues, Einstein modified into capable of provide you with the following speculation.

Space and time are the two additives of area-time, and the ensuing forces internal location-time (pressure, mass, acceleration) combine to create the phenomenon referred to as gravity. The gravity of items in vicinity-time has a warping impact on the distance-time around them, causing an ongoing push-pull inside the universe amongst devices of extra and lesser mass.

With this idea, Einstein had essentially solved one of the greatest mysteries of the universe. Prior to the discharge of his paper, "The Foundation of the General Theory of Relativity," in 1915, scientists understood what gravity modified into, however they didn't apprehend why gravity works. The exceptional manner to explain fashionable relativity is to count on that place-time is a huge sheet of fabric. If you vicinity a large item in the middle of the fabric, it will create a dip, and smaller gadgets located at the cloth will begin to roll towards the larger object. This represents the maximum essential item's gravity. But each of those smaller gadgets has its very own mass and creates its very personal small dip. Whether or no longer the ones small gadgets roll all of the manner to satisfy the large object is based upon on how an awful lot gravity they every very very own. Mass and gravity are right now related, the larger the mass, the more potent the gravity.

If the smaller item can create a dip large enough, it's going to prevent them from rolling all the way to the larger item's characteristic and help them keep their very very own place in region-time.

This is one of the motives our solar device works.

The solar continues the heaviest mass within the middle of our device, and the planets all orbit across the solar, however every is also sitting in its very very personal dip, stopping them from "rolling downhill" into the sun. There are also different forces at play that prevent the entirety from being drawn into the solar, together with man or woman rotation.

The counteraction of spin and gravity keeps each planet from leaving its orbit and being "sucked into" the solar's mass.

This additionally allows us give an explanation for the life and conduct of black holes. While our sun has a top notch amount of mass (1.989×10^{30} kg), black holes need to have a mean of three to ten times that mass. The black hole at the center of our galaxy, the Milky Way, has a mass that is 4.3 million instances that of our sun.

This indicates us why now not anything, along with light, can get away the gravity of a black hollow. Their mass is honestly too first rate compared to something else that exists within the surrounding universe. As a protracted way as Einstein's view on whether or no longer or not singularities should sign the life of wormholes for the usage of time adventure, the physicist felt that theoretically, this changed into feasible.

However, he moreover believed that if no longer some thing may additionally want to stay on being drawn into the singularity of a black hollow, then the possibilities of someone able to stay on passing via a wormhole modified into very low if no longer 0. Einstein performed a whole lot of his famous concept experiments about the possibilities of time adventure but was in no way able to postulate a concept that might be established.

General relativity additionally explains the phenomenon of time dilation, this is a few issue that takes place inner gravitational fields. Time, as we recognize or hold in mind it to be, turned into first measured hundreds of years ago. Early structures of timekeeping had been developed with the aid of the Sumerians in 3500 B.C.E., and historic Egyptian, Roman, and Greek societies additionally had structures for marking time, mainly thru using sundials. In the subsequent centuries, the invention and usage of the pendulum started out to expose that element turn out to be causally related to the every day rotation of the Earth. Eventually, the system which we recognize in recent times have emerge as subtle, that of 60 seconds to a minute, 60 minutes to an hour, and 24 hours to an afternoon.

However, Einstein favored to have the capability to reveal that aspect dilation is a real phenomenon, and he idea that his principle of extremely-contemporary relativity is probably an fantastic conduit for this concept. Time dilation takes place whilst gravity impacts now not simplest the distance round it however also the time. This can be demonstrated with a easy check here on Earth; a person who's on top of a mountain and a person within the backside of a valley can both be wearing the identical specific timekeeping device, however time will bypass quicker on pinnacle of the mountain. Why is this?

Because there can be much less gravity, the farther away you get from the center of Earth's mass.

The gravity within the valley is robust enough to simply sluggish down time.

This is the quality on-international example of time dilation.

Now, on the Earth's floor, among the valley and the mountaintop, the time dilation is perceptible however now not huge. However, if you located the idea of time dilation on a larger scale, consisting of the gravitational draw of a celebrity or a black hole, you could start to see why that is a awesome attention in Einstein's concept of giant relativity. The slowing of time close to gadgets with a dense mass and gravitational pull has implications on all items moving thru vicinity-time. It is a proscribing detail on interstellar region excursion, which we are hoping sooner or later to achieve, and explains why we see the acceleration of devices closer to gadgets with higher gravitational pull. That gravity isn't handiest affecting the rate and acceleration of the devices that it is pulling in, however that gravitational pull is likewise making time itself flow faster.

Another idea that Einstein felt modified into described thru substantial relativity is that of freefall.

We have a tendency to recall falling in normal existence as a characteristic of acceleration and gravity.

We recognise from our primary medical know-how that mass, tempo, time, and pressure can all be used to calculate how rapid some aspect will fall.

But Einstein wasn't inquisitive about classical physics and mechanics. What he preferred to discover grow to be the concept of falling with out the opposing forces of friction, gravity, and resistancein different terms, freefall.

Using the idea of famous relativity, Einstein modified into capable of conclude that absent any forces of gravity, an object can also want to theoretically fall all the time until it changed into acted upon via an outside pressure or item, mainly, landing upon a floor. Einstein hypothesized that considering the fact that each one gadgets in freefall enjoy the identical acceleration irrespective of mass whilst the gravitational pressure is the Earth-desired 9.8m/sec2, then when gravity grow to be elevated or reduced because of a warp or pulling down of place-time (don't forget our fabric instance?), then the acceleration or deceleration of freefall can also be affected.

General relativity offers lots to bite on.

But with the aid of manner of know-how actually those few vital tenets, it's clean to appearance why Einstein's theories had and still have such an impact on nearly each soar ahead in quantum physics, quantum mechanics, and theoretical physics when you take into account that.

Thinking about cutting-edge relativity in truth gives you pause to remember your place inside the universe, doesn't it?

From the tiniest particles and photons to the densest black holes, we occupy such a very specific area so that you can observe and recognize each ends of the spectrum.

Later Years and Lasting Impacts of Einstein's Work

While it can look like maximum Einstein's seminal works came while he come to be nevertheless young, the physicist loved an extended profession training, visiting, and lecturing till he exceeded away inside the United States in 1955. Like loads of his theories, Einstein's existence itself turned into complicated and marred by means of manner of warfare and personal contradictions. One of the world's maximum first-rate medical minds became not the fantastic, even via his personal admission, at interpersonal relationships. He had two marriages that were laid low with his inability to live committed. He changed into furthermore a renowned pacifist, a trait that might lend him a repeating challenge rely of moral conflicts.

As you bear in mind, Einstein renounced his beginning citizenship in the German Empire to keep away from compulsory navy issuer, turning into a Swiss citizen in 1901. In 1914, he signed an real announcement that announced to all of Europe that he changed into a pacifist and a globalist, underlining his notion that his technology belonged to absolutely everyone, now not in reality the ones of the united states of america in which he have become living and operating. At the realization of World War I, Einstein turn out to be invited to go to, excursion, and lecture within the United States for the primary time. He arrived within the US in 1921 and spent over a month using his appearances as a fundraiser for the Hebrew University in Jerusalem.

It modified into round 1926 while the two faculties of concept in quantum physics and quantum mechanics, Einstein's university and Bohr's university, started out to sincerely diverge. In 1927, the two men should have interaction in a sequence of rather well-known debates. This debate collection started out out to open up the area of physics to the general public, and Einstein's popular way of life stock began to jump all once more. The rise of the Nazi party in Germany concerned Einstein, and so he everyday a characteristic at Princeton University in New Jersey because the pinnacle of the Institute of Advanced Study. While he had meant to cut up his time between New Jersey and Berlin, his stance as a pacifist made him unwelcome in his native Germany. In 1933, he resigned from the Prussian Academy of Sciences and declared that he would possibly in all likelihood in no manner cross lower returned to his hometown.

While walking inside the United States, Einstein became painfully conscious that many awesome physicists had been difficult at paintings looking to harness nuclear strength for use in weapons. He even signed off on a letter to President Franklin D.

Roosevelt explaining that German scientists were furthermore running at the nuclear technology needed to create an atomic bomb. Although he end up deeply rooted in his private pacifism, Einstein recommended america president to make sure that the army modified into diligent in its private pursuit of nuclear weaponry. Einstein knew the significance of his art work inside the development of this era and favored to make sure the chief of his new home did as well.

Despite this, and notwithstanding becoming a United States citizen in 1940, Einstein ought to in no way art work without delay on the manufacturing of the atomic bomb. The scientists who have been part of the Manhattan Project had been expressly forbidden from speaking to Einstein because of his left-wing political leanings. Although nuclear fission ought to not have been possible with out Einstein's equation of mass equivalence, he may additionally never artwork at once with atomic weaponry, a truth which didn't hassle him inside the slightest. He knew the impact he'd already had on its improvement, however due to his deep perception that technology belongs to the people, Einstein additionally felt he had no manage over what others chose to collectively collectively together with his theories and findings.

The purpose the E=mc2, became so crucial within the advancement of nuclear era is that it gave scientists a context internal to paintings on splitting the atom. Nuclear fission is on the heart of atomic weaponry. Nuclear electricity itself is relying on the herbal decay of radioactivity, and soon the technology can be used to construct strength flowers and nuclear-powered watercraft like submarines. Mass equivalency is what allowed scientists to apprehend that they will use minimal quantities of dense radioactive elements, like uranium, to create massive amounts of energy, like a nuclear explosion. In managed settings like a energy plant, radiation from exceptionally radioactive elements is trapped because the materials decay and harnessed into electric powered energy.

In his later years, Einstein, who had normally been considered a piece of an outlier, began out to distance himself from the theories that his colleagues were supplying. He became unhappy with the path that quantum mechanics have become taking, and actively spoke out towards his antique contemporaries, even after his public debates along alongside along with his friend Niels Bohr. As Bohr have turn out to be extra entrenched in mechanics, their critiques and faculties of notion need to in no manner pass all another time. It end up Heisenberg's assertion that the "quantum revolution" became over that sent Einstein firmly and with finality on foot from the set up order.

Although Einstein's critical accomplishments all happened earlier than 1930, he in no way as soon as stopped strolling on developing new theories, writing papers, and lecturing. He published loads of quick works amongst 1930 and his demise in 1955 and renewed his Jewish religion. He turned into even provided the presidency of the younger Jewish sovereign united states of america of Israel in 1952. At the time of his passing in 1955, he committed all his time and research to growing what he referred to as a "unified concern principle," which he believed is probably the grasp key to unlocking all of quantum, classical, and mechanical physics. While he wasn't a success in solidifying this speculation earlier than his demise, he might be happy to apprehend he kickstarted a advertising and marketing advertising marketing campaign that continues nowadays to discover the so-called "precept of the whole thing."

Chapter 7: A Glimpse Into The Future Of Quantum Take A Look At

Although the smooth premises of quantum physics were set through the mid-1900s, that doesn't advise that the advances made through the pioneers of the sector stopped there. Scientists keep to artwork each day to liberate new and thrilling theories about the conduct of atoms, particles, and waves. Our ever-growing statistics of those unseen topics is what brings us some of the generation we enjoy in our ordinary lives.

Think approximately the topics you probable did while to procure up this morning. Without the pioneers of energy, you would had been in a position to turn at the slight and begin your coffeepot.

Without the scientists who decided microwaves, you wouldn't be able to warmness up your breakfast, and your mobile phone wouldn't exist without electric powered engineers and quantum physicists. Our lives might be completely one in all a type if we didn't have a number of the maximum incredible scientific minds furiously advancing the field of quantum have a take a look at within the early part of the 20 th century.

The exquisite issue is, we've got the equal shape of terrific minds these days who preserve to increase our knowledge of quantum conduct.

There are experiments going on international in limitless laboratories which may be finding new topics at a breakneck pace.

In the later a part of the 2oth century, huge branches of take a look at started to emerge among those quantum scientists who wanted to hold to have a take a look at the tiny things atoms, subatomic debris, photons, and quarks. These scientists and mathematicians are operating little by little to recognize and classify the conduct of the maximum infinitesimal elements of preserve in mind.

The 2d university of quantum physicists is those who need to apply what's mentioned approximately the tiniest matters to the largest matters planets, stars, galaxies, and all the special bodies, visible and unseen, that make up the greater universe.

Astrophysicists may don't have whatever to have a look at if it weren't for particle physicists. Being capable of count on the behavior of an atom technique that we're capable of exchange the conduct of the entirety that's product of atoms.

Similarly, a deep expertise of wave conduct manner understanding what to anticipate from waves of all sizes, wavelengths, and styles of keep in mind, in conjunction with gravitational waves. Let's have a have a look at what's taking region these days in each fields.

Quantum Mechanics in the

21st Century

There are some regions of attention in the examine of quantum mechanics in the twenty first century.

The first and most famous is the existence of the Higgs bosun, which end up examined to be confirmed through experiments being run on the Large Hadron Collider at CERN in Switzerland in 2012.

This become the cease result of a few years of observe of the components which make up debris. Over the course of the mid to overdue20th century, scientists were able to determine that even protons, electrons, and neutrons had been crafted from even smaller quantities, and the Higgs boson was one of the most elusive.

Another place of quantum mechanics that current physicists are trying to training session is that of quantum entanglement. This is a conundrum which means that once in a while, the houses of one quantum substance can't be superb from the houses of each other due to the truth the materials or gadgets are "entangled" interior a gadget. Despite understanding that there are top notch devices with their personal trends within the device, a scientist want to check the behavior of every substances which will have a take a look at one. The substances should be described at the issue of each one of a kind, or the observations might be defective.

One distinctive primary focus location of quantum mechanics is on quantum computing (the usage of arithmetic to are searching forward to the conduct of micro-quantum particles, like quarks and bosuns) and quantum transfers, that is the movement of records and depend the usage of quantum-stage communications. This is surely the stuff of technological expertise fiction due to the fact the surrender result may additionally want to ultimately be the switch of big rely debris the usage of wave mechanics and quantum particle movement.

Of direction, we are despite the fact that years or some years some distance from being transported from vicinity to location, as is depicted in famous sci-fi shows and movies, but it's drastically a laugh to consider.

Of course, there is that entire pesky difficulty about not being able to be put returned together well, but all in appropriate time.

Those who study quantum mechanics moreover maintain to growth their data of wave conduct, which has a right away effect on normal life in the 21st century. Broadband communications and increasingly more fast and reliable mobile cell smartphone networks are one incredible gain of the art work of wave mechanic scientists. So too are the additives that pass into our communique and entertainment gadgets. Being capable of construct receivers and transponders that can manipulate swiftly evolving transmission tool is equally crucial.

Quantum mechanics is also answerable for most of the opportunity topics we're all acquainted with lasers, atomic clocks, pc structures, and MRI technology.

Even the era that goes into things like satellite tv for laptop television for pc dishes and sun panels is all way to quantum mechanics and a critical expertise of ways debris and waves art work.

One of the most sizable improvements inside the last hundred years become the development of the electron microscope a present to scientists from scientists.

As folks who examine quantum mechanics retain to boom their records and knowledge of the mechanical motion of the universe's tiniest debris, you can most effective consider the advances that we are capable of see over the subsequent a long term and centuries.

Quantum Physics within the

twenty first Century

Quantum physics is indelibly related to quantum mechanics, however while a few scientists choose to cognizance their energies on analyzing the infinitesimal particle this is the idea of all quantum studies, some choose out to take a look at the huge photo. Many quantum physicists nowadays spend time studying and re-studying Einstein's theories and workout them on the manner to take a look at the universe at big.

The improvement of location exploration and our deepening know-how of place is essentially in detail to Einstein's theories of relativity. Whether it's miles the era this is going into big telescopes that help us see the outer reaches of our solar gadget or galaxy or the inner workings of manned location flight, none of these items will be viable if Einstein didn't supply the arena the manner through which to every positioned the ones devices and those in place and interpret the results in their research.

Einstein's information of the behavior of rely quantity and his clarification of the character of gravity have been instrumental in being able to study the universe past the confines of Earth. The precept of ultra-modern relativity elements into nearly the entirety about space tour and exploration; it's moreover an first-rate possibility for scientists and astronauts to preserve to prove those theories right. From having the ability to tell if radio transmission waves are bending to house gravitational fields to being capable of decide if planets are orbiting a long way flung stars, the concept of fashionable relativity is normally being utilized in area.

Quantum physics also accomplished a big feature in being able to take the first actual image of a black hollow, which befell in 2017. This become groundbreaking paintings for masses obvious reasons, however it is also one of the best symptoms that Einstein's idea literally holds real universally. The photo, taken over a length of five days the use of a sequence of 8 telescopes in a worldwide-massive collaboration, indicates a huge fuel cloud surrounding a black hollow this is 54 mild-years faraway from Earth.

A black hole is a acquainted region object, but one that we might also in no manner understand the appropriate nature of, and that's due to the fact its severe gravitational pull makes it nearly not viable to apprehend what occurs "inner" the black hollow itself. Modern quantum physicists and astrophysicists conflict to reconcile the data they have, the information they want, and the expertise they will in no way benefit. This doesn't prevent the ones scientists from running tirelessly to recognize the mysteries of the universe.

One essential quandary that faces quantum physicists is that ever because of the fact that the schools of notion cut up among Bohr and Einstein, it has been tough to return to grips with the reality that the 2 fundamentals of quantum studiesmechanics and relativityare basically at odds with each particular. Both camps maintain to find out new reasons of approaches the universe works, however neither can truly agree with the alternative. Those who are going for walks inside the fields of relativity can, but, agree that there will always be new worlds and new rely to find out.

One such manner that those scientists preserve Einstein's legacy alive is through attempting to reveal the existence of darkish keep in mind and dark strength. We recognise that count and energy are identical, and we apprehend that rely and strength can't be created or destroyed. But there are unseen forces inside the universe that could first-class be explained through way of the presence of power and rely than we're but to recognize. So, what are darkish count number and darkish electricity, and what are scientists doing to attempt to understand it?

In smooth phrases, dark depend is what remains after the identified depend inside the universe is accounted for.

This depend may be product of black holes, brown dwarves, or other dense, colorless do not forget, even though it's probable we would be capable of see or stumble on the presence of such big or mass-dense devices. It's moreover theorized that dark keep in mind range is made from the alternative of the debris that we're acquainted with, despite the truth that the idea of anti-depend is more likely despite the fact that the purview of generation fiction. It's most probable that darkish remember, which makes up approximately 75-80% of the diagnosed universe, is a aggregate of but-to-be-identified quantum particles, undetected black holes, and one-of-a-type dense neutron stars.

The maximum uninteresting and maximum in all likelihood solution, no matter the truth that, is that darkish rely is crafted from the identical atoms and molecules as appeared do not forget; we sincerely haven't been able to see it but.

Dark electricity is every one of a kind story.

Dark strength is the stress that looks to be causing the universe to be ever-growing, and nobody has quite figured it out but. We recognise that darkish energy exists. We recognize that it is at the back of the growth of the universe, and we also recognize that it's inflicting that increase to enhance up. What we don't apprehend about dark energy is why it's miles doing this. For some time, astrophysicists had been involved that this rapid growth should advocate that the universe became jogging its manner in the direction of self-destructionthat like an elastic constructing up potential electricity as it is stretched, it'd in the long run virtually snap lower again. This ought to reason the alternative of the Big Bang and has been dubbed the Big Crunch.

Now scientists view the persevering with, quickening growth of the universe as more of an infinite behavior. That no matter the truth that we recognize that don't forget and power can't be created or destroyed, the universe will subsequently need to put on itself out, and the boom will each save you, or the universe will pop like a balloon. Thankfully, we received't have to don't forget any of these occasions happening in our lifetime, but physicists are although running to discover solutions as to why dark take into account and dark power have such an effect on the diagnosed universe. The more solutions they may be able to gain, the better hazard anyone have of knowledge the workings of all the take into account we can not see.

On a happier observe, than the eventual destruction of the universe, quantum physicists are strolling in new strategies to endure in mind the ranges of depend, and manned location flight gives them the opportunity to gain this. Trained astronauts at the International Space Station have get right of entry to to the vacuum of place to carry out experiments on sublimation and condensation, in addition to see how the distance vacuum impacts the ionization of pretty some factors.

Another benefit of getting the capability to test theories and substances in the environs and vacuum of place is being privy to a 0-gravity environment.

Under the ones situations, the forces of gravity can't have an impact on the particles that astronauts are reading.

Many of the individuals who now adventure to the International Space Station to work are knowledgeable scientists who took on the extra burden of becoming astronauts, whereas, in lots of years beyond, it became scientists on Earth who might train astronauts on a manner to behave as their studies proxies at the identical time as in region. The end result is a cross-professional vicinity contingent who're constantly attempting out the bounds of the behavior of be counted range every nearby to area and brought to that surroundings.

Scientists who art work in observatories and at region businesses are constantly looking for new techniques to gain more data of the workings of the universe, which incorporates studies into the origins of depend, whether or now not the charge of mild in fact is the ordinary pace restriction, and if there are new and interesting strategies to apply Einstein's standards to "see" beyond the outer stretches of region with the beneficial aid of detecting new gravitational fields. No rely what the future holds, we can all relaxation assured that physicists are going for walks tough to assist us understand the very nature of the distance we occupy, on each a tiny scale and a regularly going on one.

We've now come close to to the quit of our time together, and it's been a heck of a adventure through time to take a look at physics!

Before you get to the perception of the ebook, you'll locate appendices, which can be meant to help you recap and bear in mind the thoughts we protected. The first appendix is a timeline of early physics breakthroughs and discoveries, and the second one is a listing of components and equations at the way to be of use to you in case you need to start crunching numbers to your very non-public.

There are so many one-of-a-kind fields that erupted from the identical antique beginnings of classical physics.

If you're inquisitive about how the area works, you then sincerely are inquisitive about physics.

But with a panoply of options, if you've determined that quantum physics isn't for you, then congrats!

At least you made it all of the way through the e-book before you made a decision that. Maybe you'd like to check out quantum mechanics, quantum statistics, or quantum electromagnetics. Perhaps you're more inclined to fall into the classical mechanics camp, in which you may have a look at thermodynamics, mechanical wave precept, or classical statistics.

If you like to dabble inside the unknown, you can want to discover the sector of theoretical physics. You also can need to hypothesize about black holes, string principle, wormholes, and time tour. The global dreams greater dreamers who're inclined to again up their desires with technological know-how. Many of the sector's coolest and maximum loved enhancements had been created thru scientists who dared to dream, so possibly you can be the subsequent. No rely in which you are for your existence or in which you want your science journey to take you, actually do not forget that there's no incorrect desire whilst you pick out to check era.

Humans are innately curious beings, and our functionality for higher idea and reasoning is what gadgets us apart from the relaxation of the animal u . S .. We may additionally want to theorize, carry out the medical method, and gain answers through notion, movement, terms, and numbers. For all aspiring scientists, that is a comforting concept. Although atoms and debris are small, and the universe is big, we are able to continuously take coronary coronary heart that technology is concrete and acquired't lead us off track.

We desire you cherished analyzing your way thru the basics of quantum physics and which you've been inspired to take your scientific expertise to the subsequent stage!

Chapter 8: The Birth Of Quantum Mechanics

The start of quantum mechanics marks a pivotal moment inside the records of physics, because it represents a important shift in our information of the behavior of depend and power at the smallest scales. The journey to quantum mechanics changed into a tumultuous one, characterized by using using groundbreaking discoveries and profound paradigm shifts.

Early Pioneers: Planck and Einstein

The origins of quantum mechanics can be traced decrease lower lower back to the past due 19th and early 20th centuries at the same time as physicists had been grappling with the mysteries of atomic and subatomic phenomena. Max Planck performed a vital function in starting up this revolution. In 1900, he brought the idea of quantization of power to offer an reason for the spectrum of blackbody radiation. Planck proposed that electricity turn out to be quantized into discrete packets, or "quanta," in choice to being continuously disbursed. This grows to be an intensive departure from classical physics.

Albert Einstein in addition advanced the ones ideas in 1905 even as he defined the photoelectric impact. He recommended that slight consists of discrete packets of power, which we now call photons. This idea now not satisfactory supported Planck's quantization but moreover challenged the prevailing wave idea of light.

Wave-Particle Duality

One of the essential aspect dispositions within the delivery of quantum mechanics become the recognition of wave-particle duality. This concept, which received prominence within the early 20th century, posits that debris which includes electrons and photons display off both wave-like and particle-like conduct counting on how they are located. This duality shattered the classical belief of fantastic debris following particular trajectories.

CHALLENGES TO CLASSICAL PHYSICS

The begin of quantum mechanics have become driven through a sequence of experimental effects that couldn't be defined via way of classical physics. Phenomena similar to the quantization of atomic power degrees and the remark of discrete spectral strains in atomic spectra challenged the deterministic worldview of classical mechanics.

These worrying conditions brought about the improvement of a new mathematical framework to explain the behavior of debris at the quantum diploma. Werner Heisenberg, Erwin Schrödinger, and others done pivotal roles in formulating the mathematical formalism of quantum mechanics.

Schrödinger's Equation

In 1926, Erwin Schrödinger brought his famous wave equation, referred to as

Schrödinger's equation. This equation offers a mathematical description of the quantum kingdom of a gadget and how it evolves over time. It laid the foundation for information the behavior of quantum particles and remains a primary detail of quantum mechanics to at the prevailing time.

The begin of quantum mechanics represented a profound shift in our statistics of the bodily world, emphasizing the probabilistic nature of quantum systems and hard classical determinism. It opened the door to a latest generation of exploration and discovery, in which the quantum world's weird and counterintuitive phenomena could probable turn out to be the focal point of clinical inquiry.

QUANTUM MECHANICS FUNDAMENTALS

Quantum mechanics, frequently called quantum physics, is a complex and fashionable theory that governs the conduct of count and energy at the smallest scales of the universe. To draw close to the essence of quantum mechanics, one must understand numerous key fundamentals that underlie this charming area of physics.

Wave Functions and Probability

Central to quantum mechanics is the idea of the wave characteristic, denoted with the useful resource of the photo Ψ (Psi). The wave feature describes the quantum country of a particle, which encompass an electron, and carries information approximately its function, momentum, and special houses. However, the wave function represents possibilities in region of certainties. The square of the absolute rate of the wave characteristic^2) offers the possibility density of locating the particle in a specific u . S . A ..

In essence, quantum mechanics offers a probabilistic framework for predicting the behavior of particles, replacing the deterministic outlook of classical physics.

The Uncertainty Principle

Werner Heisenberg's Uncertainty Principle is a cornerstone of quantum mechanics. It states that there are inherent limits to how exactly we're able to simultaneously understand high excellent pairs of homes of a particle, which encompass its role and momentum. The greater because it should be we apprehend this type of homes, the a good deal a good deal much less because it have to be we are able to realize the opportunity. This crucial dilemma demanding situations our classical intuition and underscores the probabilistic nature of quantum structures.

QUANTUM STATES AND SUPERPOSITION

Quantum mechanics introduces the idea of quantum states, which describe the viable conditions or configurations of a quantum machine. A terrific property of quantum states is superposition, wherein a particle can exist in a linear mixture of a couple of states concurrently. This approach that until measured or placed, a particle may be in multiple positions or states without delay.

Superposition is exemplified with the useful resource of manner of the famous belief take a look at regarding Schrödinger's cat, this is concurrently alive and dead till an remark collapses the cat's country into one of the opportunities.

Quantum Mechanical Model

Schrödinger's equation is the crucial equation of quantum mechanics. It describes how the wave feature of a quantum tool modifications over time. This equation allows physicists to calculate and assume the chances of various results whilst a size is made on a quantum gadget.

Quantum mechanics moreover introduces the idea of quantum operators, such as the area operator and the momentum operator, which represent bodily observables in quantum systems. These operators act on the wave characteristic to yield measurable consequences.

Understanding the ones quantum mechanics fundamentals is essential for exploring the quantum worldwide. They offer the theoretical basis for describing the conduct of particles on the quantum diploma, in which classical physics not applies. These thoughts shape the concept for the awesome phenomena and generation that have emerged from the have a take a look at of quantum mechanics.

THE QUANTUM MECHANICAL MODEL

The quantum mechanical model, furthermore known as the quantum version or quantum precept, is a essential framework in physics that gives an extensive description of the behavior of debris at the quantum diploma. It represents a departure from classical physics, as it consists of the probabilistic and wave-like nature of debris, supplying a more correct and whole information of the microcosmic global.

Schrödinger's Equation

At the coronary coronary coronary heart of the quantum mechanical model is Schrödinger's equation. Erwin Schrödinger formulated this equation in 1926, and it's far a essential equation in quantum mechanics. Schrödinger's equation describes how the quantum country of a system adjustments with time. It is a partial differential equation that operates on the wave characteristic (Ψ), it surely is a mathematical function that incorporates records about the quantum system.

Wave Functions and Probability

Wave functions (Ψ) are applicable to the quantum mechanical version. These mathematical talents describe the quantum us of a of a particle or a device of debris. The square of the absolute fee of the wave characteristicΨprobability density of locating a particle in a specific kingdom or function. In one-of-a-type words, the wave function gives statistics approximately the chance of diverse consequences whilst measurements are made on a quantum system.

Quantization of Energy

One of the profound outcomes of the quantum mechanical version is the quantization of energy ranges. In quantum structures, energy isn't always non-prevent but alternatively quantized, which means it's miles available in discrete, exceptional values. This concept is obvious in phenomena which embody the quantized electricity ranges of electrons in atoms, which offer upward push to the discrete spectral lines located in atomic spectra.

Operators and Observables

Quantum mechanics introduces the concept of operators, which can be mathematical constructs representing physical observables like function, momentum, and angular momentum. These operators act at the wave characteristic to yield measurable consequences. For example, the placement operator applied to the wave characteristic offers records about the location of a particle.

Superposition and Entanglement

Two exceptional capabilities of the quantum mechanical version are superposition and entanglement. Superposition lets in particles to exist in a combination of more than one states simultaneously until measured or determined. Entanglement, but, is a phenomenon in which the quantum states of or greater particles emerge as correlated in this sort of manner that the dimensions of one particle right away impacts the kingdom of each other, no matter the space among them.

The quantum mechanical model has induced profound insights into the conduct of particles and has paved the way for the improvement of quantum era, which encompass quantum computing and quantum cryptography. It demanding situations our classical intuitions and has improved our facts of the universe at its most vital diploma, organising the door to new discoveries and enhancements.